The Impact of a Deadly Pandemic on Individual, Society, Economy and the World

ROBERT DUPREY, PH.D.

The Impact of a Deadly Pandemic on Individual, Society, Economy and the World

Order this book online at www.trafford.com
or email orders@trafford.com

Most Trafford titles are also available at major online book retailers.

Print information available on the last page.

ISBN: 978-1-6987-0361-9 (sc)
ISBN: 978-1-6987-0360-2 (e)

Trafford rev. 10/13/2020

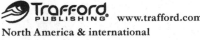 www.trafford.com

North America & international
toll-free: 844-688-6899 (USA & Canada)
fax: 812 355 4082

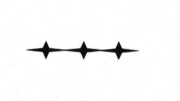

Contents

THE IMPACT OF A DEADLY PANDEMIC ON INDIVIDUAL, SOCIETY, ECONOMY AND THE WORLD

Introduction

Viruses have changed the quality of our life and our society drastically in many ways. The Coronavirus pandemic has caused global and social disruption as we have seen it in 2020 and created the largest global recession since the Great Depression. It has led to the postponement or cancellation of businesses, shopping centers, sporting, religious, political, and cultural events worldwide, widespread supply shortages exacerbated by panic buying (The New York Times News,

2020). Schools, universities, and colleges have been closed either on a nationwide level or local level in 177 countries, affecting approximately 98.6% of the world's student population (Unesco, 2020). On the other hand it decreased emissions of pollutants and reduction in greenhouse gases and this is the only positive results from 2019-2020 Covid-19 pandemic.

There are seven types of Human Coronavirus that infected humans. 1) **HCoV-OC43**, 2) **HC0V-229E**, 3) **HCoV-NL63**, 4) **HCoV-HKU1** each with length of immunity of 1 to 2 years and 5) **MERS-CoV**, 6) **SARS-CoV** and finally 7) **SARS-CoV-2** with unclear length of immunity. 1) **HCoV-OC43** infected human and cattle, 2) **HCoV-229E** infected humans and bats, 3) **HCoV-NL63** infected mostly young children and the elderly, 4) **HCoV-HKU1** was discovered in Hong Kong China and was related to the Mouse Hepatitis Virus (MHV), 5) **MERS-CoV** was discovered in Saudi Arabia in 2012 and infected all Middle Eastern countries, 6) **SARS-CoV** was discovered in South China and the virus was transferred to human from wild animals sold as food in local market in many reigns of China, 7) **SARS-CoV-2** known as Covid-19 (COrona VIrus Disease of 2019) that caused the worldwide outbreak discovered in China. It is assumed that this virus was emerged from bat-borne virus and transferred to humans. The scientific consensus was that similar to the family of Coronaviruses (mentioned above) the Covid-19 has also a natural origin. The name was given by the World Health Organization (WHO) for the virus. The probable bat-to-human infection may have been among people processing bat carcasses and guano in the production of traditional Chinese medicines (Letters in Applied Microbiology, 2020). Bats and other wild animals are being sold as food in many parts of China at present time.

These viruses are zoonotic, meaning that they commonly infect animals and can transfer to humans.

There was a rumor about the Covid-19 pandemic sensitivity to temperature. Current evidence shows that while the Covid-19 appears to be stable at low and freezing temperatures for a certain period. Regardless of the climate, the virus can be transmitted in any climate and there is no solid evidence to believe that cold or hot weather can kill the virus. There are many medical details that are unknown for this virus. Sometimes wrong information or misinformation and lack of transparency in addition to lack of data and facts from the source have caused spread of rumors through social media and medical news media.

Many countries including the U.S. have blamed China for failing to take precautionary measures to stop the virus quickly from spreading globally and killing thousands. In respond to that there have been incidents of discrimination against Chinese people and against those perceived as being Chinese or as being from areas with high infection rates (Tavernise S, Oppel Jr, 2020). It is believed that the virus will be around for years to come even if the Corona vaccine is developed.

The question is; can anyone catch Coronavirus twice? A new study of people who have caught and recovered from Coronavirus raises the prospect that immunity to the virus may be short-lived. Scientists found that levels of antibodies faded over a three (3) months period. According to BBC News "This may have a big impact on how the world copes with the virus in the future. This is also why the World Health Organization (WHO) is nervous about countries using immunity passports as a way out of lockdown. Swipe through for more on the issue of virus immunity". In spite of all this, the Coronavirus pandemic may never goes away, even with a vaccine. It is very possible having new and more powerful viruses much deadlier than the Covid-19 in the future. The threat for nuclear attack is less likely than biological attach.

In this book the writer will examine the impact of the Coronavirus pandemic on individual, society, economy, workplace and the globe, and what governments of different countries can do in order to successfully defeat the pandemic and other similar killer viruses of the future. Finally the writer will define a safer workplace for the future and a better Society for next generation and will proposed solutions on how to safely control the pandemic.

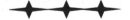

Background

It has been more than six months since the World Health Organization (WHO) declared the Coronavirus threat a pandemic. The virus is continuing its spread across the world with nearly 30 million confirmed cases in 188 countries and a death toll fast approaching one million.

On 31 December 2019, health authorities in China reported to the World Health Organization (WHO) a cluster of viral pneumonia cases of unknown virus in Wuhan, Hubei China and an investigation was launched in early January 2020 (BBC News, 2020). On 30 January 2020, the WHO and Public Health Emergency of International Concern (PHEIC) declared the outbreak with a total number of 6,065 confirmed cases globally. By mid-September 2020 more than 30,290,791 cases confirmed globally and close to 947,919 were dead worldwide. The highest death toll caused by the pandemic was the U.S. and the total deaths estimated 200,000+ by mid-September of 2020.

Several of the early infected cases of the Coronavirus had visited Huanan seafood wholesale market in China and it is believed that the virus was thought to have a zoonotic origin and to some degree of bat to human infection. Some believed this virus has been developed in lab by Chinese and the President Trump called it "Chinese Virus" and distributed in Huanan seafood wholesale market. Either way, the origin of both SARS and the Covid-19 known to be China. This might have been an intentional attempt to down fall the global economy and the effect of it in the U.S. 2020 presidential election.

The earliest known person with symptoms was later discovered to have fallen ill on 1 December 2019, and that person did not have visible connections with the later wet market cluster. Of the early cluster of cases reported that month, two-thirds (2/3) of the people in Wuhan China were found to have a link with the seafood wholesale market (Chan JF, Yuan S, Kok KH, To KK, Chu H, Yang J, 2020). On 13 March 2020, an unverified report from the South China Morning Post suggested; a case traced back to 17 November 2019 (a 55-year-old person from Hubei China) may have been the first person infected (SCMP, 2020).

The WHO (World Health Organization) recognized the spread of the Covid-19 as a pandemic on 11 March 2020. Italy, Iran, South Korea, and Japan reported high surging cases. The total numbers of cases outside China quickly passed China's. (gisanddata.maps.arcgis.com, 2020).

The Covid-19 pandemic has caused so much disruption to the economy and non-coronavirus medical care that it is upending the outlook for next year's employer health coverage. Insurers cannot forecast how much elective surgical care will rebound in the second half of 2020. With rising infection rates in southern and western states of the U.S, which could spook patients to continue to postpone care until end of 2021. More than two (2) million people worldwide have died from the virus, with the U.S. reporting more deaths and infections from Covid-19 than any other nation, according to tallies by Johns Hopkins University (Sept 2020).

The Trump administration has hinted for months that the U.S. would take steps to punish China for failing to prevent the deadly virus, which was first observed in the Chinese city of Wuhan, from spreading around the globe. According to the United States Secretary State Mike Pompeo (2020) "the world will make China pay a price for the unfolding global health pandemic caused by the coronavirus. I am very confident that the world will look at China differently and engage with them fundamentally different than they did before this catastrophic disaster". President Donald Trump signed legislation to impose sanctions on China in response to its interference with Hong Kong's autonomy.

According to CNBC the Trump administration accused China of working with the World Health Organization to downplay the growing coronavirus crisis and withdrew from the World Health Organization on July 6, 2020. Pompeo said "The result today is that we have hundreds of thousands of people who have died and trillions of dollars in global damage as a direct result of the Chinese Communist Party's decision". The U.S. has reported an average of about 62,210 new cases per day over seven days in July 2020, up more than

21% compared with the seven-day average weeks back in July, according to a CNBC analysis of the data from Hopkins. The U.S. conducted 760,282 tests in July 2020, the second-highest number of tests conducted in a single day, according to data compiled by the Covid Tracking Project.

The nuclear atomic bomb in 1945 had killed more than 150,000 people in one day in Hiroshima Japan. Coronavirus has killed more than 600,000 in 3 months worldwide in 2020. It is estimated this number to double by the end of 2021.

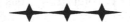

Impact on Individual

Massive unemployment that was caused by the Coronavirus in 2020 has left deep scars not only in the U.S. but worldwide. According to The Guardian (2020), Last count of worldwide unemployment exceeded far more in 2020 than before and this number estimated to triple.

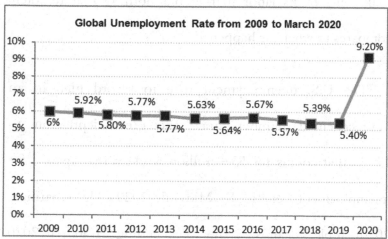

Source: www.oecd.org/economic-outlook/june-2020/

40,000 workers filed for unemployment benefits in the USA in May of 2020. This number most likely to triple during the course of this pandemic by the end of 2021 and beyond and more workers will be forced to unemployment and loss of income. This will cause spare time for lots of workers forcing them to stay home more than any other period of modern history. The surge in unemployment in the United States caused by the pandemic shattered all previous records. In its time, the world's biggest economy has seen some savage shake-outs of its labor market but nothing that remotely compares to what has happened.

The U.S. unemployment rose to record high in an unprecedented number since the great depression to 15.2% that counts for 53+ million workers that applied for unemployment benefits by Mid July 2020 (The Guardian, 2020). Jobless claims in the week ending 21 March 2020 surged to almost 3.3 million, which was double what Wall

Street analysts had collectively been expecting (The Guardian,

2020). The previous total unemployment in October 1982

was just one fifth (1/5) of the said level. Before the pandemic

struck, the U.S. had its lowest unemployment rate since the

late 1960s. That is now history. The official jobless rate was

about to rocket from just under 4% to at least 20% to 30% if

the economy with the pandemic still lingering in 2020 stays

the same. Rising unemployment has not been helpful to sitting

U.S. president seeking re-election, which perhaps explains

why the U.S. government's stimulus package contained more

generous benefits for those losing their jobs and that might

be the reason that Donald Trump was so keen to get the

economy going again and he called on supporters to "liberate"

states that have experienced protests over Coronavirus

lockdowns right a day after he unveiled guidelines aimed at

reopening the nation's economy (Patriot Journal, 2020).

The mental and physical stresses caused by fear of layoff have left many individuals feeling suicidal. Unemployment and the risk of being made unemployed make people miserable. There has been plenty of speculation in the past about whether the lockdown has been good for levels of wellbeing, but the survey evidence and the economic analysts suggest it has not. According to The Guardian "11% of unemployed people who have experienced stress during the pandemic nothing had helped them to cope with the worry and anxiety" (The Guardian, 2020).

In information age that we are in, more sophisticated software technologies are bringing civilization ever closer to near workless and office-less world. Technology companies such as Facebook, Instagram, Amazon and all other similar multi-media in the USA are getting richer and richer because of the Pandemic. Companies like Zoom or Google Hangouts are examples of a new Silicon Valley startup focusing on a consumer product inspired by the coronavirus pandemic. Similar companies are taking advantage of the Covid-19 situation to provide products in mass communication and multimedia platforms. That is due to the fact that individuals are isolated and they are utilizing online purchases through Amazon.com. Interconnectivity between family members is more than ever through social media software platforms because of the pandemic. There are some people, who were sailing through the pandemic lockdown untroubled, but many have lost their jobs or they have laid-off. Others who are small business owners feel responsible for the livelihoods of others relay on them. Some have the luxury of working from home on full pay or those who collect retirement benefits or pension but the fact is that lots of people don't have money to bring food to the table because of the pandemic.

The work of economists such as Danny Blanchflower (2004) and Andrew Oswald (1994) has highlighted how higher unemployment is, as the economic variable, most strikingly linked to rising unhappiness, and the longer the spell of unemployment the greater the cost to personal well-being.

A decade's worth of job gains wiped out in just matter of weeks in 2020. Minorities, women and Hispanic American were among those who suffered the most. They, however, have contributed to the growth of the U.S. economy in recent years but because of the pandemic Hispanic Americans were the highest unemployment rate in April 2020, a major blow to Latino after achieving economic gains and before the pandemic. According to The Guardian "The jobs report also unveiled the grim reality of which communities have been hit the hardest from the economic impacts of the pandemic Hispanic Americans saw the highest unemployment rate of any racial group at 18.9%, over 4% more than the national

unemployment rate of 14.7%". Hispanic American families

are more likely to be in poverty than white families, with 17%

of Hispanic families in poverty in 2018 compared to 10% of

white families (The Guardian, 2020).

According to HuffPost (September 2020) In April 2020 and

at the start of the COVID-19 shutdown, the jobless rate was a

record-high 14.7%. In September 2020, the Labor Department

announced that the unemployment rate had dropped to 8.4%,

but digging deeper into the jobs report, it was discovered that

nearly all the improvement in the unemployment rate over the

past few months in 2020 had been for white workers. The Black

unemployment rate is still in double digits at 13%. The rate for

white workers is 7.3%, nearly half of what it is for Black workers.

In other words, white workers were getting hired back nearly twice

as fast as Black workers and Black people are getting left behind.

Here are some stats analyzing the impact of the pandemic in the USA in May 2020 (Source: The Guardian 2020):

— U.S. national unemployment rate: 14.7%

— U.S. black unemployment rates: 16.7%

— U.S Hispanic unemployment rates: 18.9%

— Percentage of unemployed Americans women: 55%

— U.S. leisure and hospitality unemployment rate: 39.8%

— U.S. state with the highest unemployment rate: Nevada

— U.S. average unemployment insurance benefit amount: about $980

— U.S. highest number of unemployment claims in one week in May 2020: 6.6 million

— U.S. number of households deemed food insecure: 1 in 5

— U.S. number of gig workers unemployed: more than 6.1million

— U.S. percentage of low-wage workers unemployed: 40%

According to the Centers for Disease Control and Prevention (CDC) of those killed by covid-19 more than 75% have been Hispanic, Black and American Indian children, even though they represent 41% of the U.S. population. One key factor could be underlying health disparities among minority children and young adults. About 75% of those who died had at least one underlying condition and the most frequent were asthma and obesity and these two conditions that disproportionately occur in the U.S. minority youths.

According to The Guardian (2020) Outside of politicians, some small businesses who are struggling to hire African American workers have complained that their employees would not return to work because they are making more on unemployment. This is a particular concern because businesses to qualify for government's PPP (Paycheck

Protection Program) forgiveness loan were to encourage keeping staff on payroll, and companies must spend 75% on payroll. For many small business owners "All of a sudden, for the first time in many business owners' lives, they were day-to-day, they were literally one day at a time in 2020, when the pandemic started coming in," (The Guardian, 2020). The people who stand to benefit the most from the boost of stimulate programs are those in the hardest-hit industries, such as healthcare workers (non-Medical doctors), food & medical delivery personal, janitors and healthcare drivers, where wages were already low. Women and other low wage workers making minimum wage are also people facing uncertainty about when and how many jobs will be available once the economy opens up.

The U.S. small businesses rehire staff but cut pay and hours, survey finds. Worker headcount among small businesses is nearly back to pre-Covid-19 levels, according to exclusive data from human resource provider Gusto (July, 2020). However, employees are now working reduced hours and with lower pay. At this point, many business owners have used the bulk of the loans they received from the federal Paycheck Protection Program (PPP) and have exhausted that money in few weeks. Meantime, large employers are unsure about the economy and whether they will need to make more job cuts, are taking longer to lock in commitments for next year.

As we reckon with what the post-Covid world looked like, we cannot forget who kept our country running in our moment of need. "Our healthcare workers, food-service workers and janitors, who are overwhelmingly African American and Hispanic American workers, women and immigrants, deserve more than praise. They deserve nothing less than family-sustaining wages of at least $15 an hour

and the right to form a union to lift up individuals and

communities, both now and in the post-pandemic world."

(The Guardian, 2020

Many individuals have lost their jobs and with that they

lost their sense of well-being, not motivated to do good

things, lost interest on daily activities, and most definitely

have used up their credit line to the max to pay bills because

of unemployment. Other groups of individuals have not

been able to pay monthly bills for at least six (6) months and

defaulted on their houses, cars and other big household items.

It is estimated that average U.S. family credit cards debt is

around $25,000 before the pandemic and $50,000 post-

pandemic. There will be overwhelming number of defaults on

houses and foreclosures in 2021 and 2022 in the U.S. because

of unemployment and lack of income very similar to 2008

financial crisis and all is due to the pandemic. It is estimated that the U.S. individual bankruptcies will be record high in the history of the U.S.A.

Other groups of individuals have been more creative and they used their spare time at home to build home-made masks, learning to cook gourmet foods, compose music, teach kids, and grow plants and build many other useful items. On the other hand, violence and abuse has been raised during the pandemic both inside and outside home. Physical abuse, child abuse, drug abuse and domestic violence has been record high during the pandemic and that is due to the fact that men and women are spending more time together under one roof for a long time isolated and unable to socialize with others and that sometimes causes family issues and domestic violence. On 5 April 2020, the united nation Secretary-General called for "a global ceasefire and an end to all violence everywhere so that we can focus our attention and resources on stopping the pandemic". Domestic violence against women and has been increasing globally as the Covid-19 pandemic combines with economic and social stresses and measures to restrict contact and movement. Crowded homes, substance abuse, limited access to services and reduced peer support are exacerbating these conditions.

According to UN report (April 2020), "Before the pandemic, it was estimated that one in three women will experience violence during their lifetimes and many of these women are trapped in their homes with their abusers". At the same time, support services are struggling. Judicial, police and health services that are the first responders for women are overwhelmed with the pandemic and have shifted priorities, or are otherwise unable to help. Civil society groups are affected by lockdown or reallocation of resources. Some domestic violence shelters are full and others have had to close or have been repurposed as health centers. All these issues are due to the pandemic. It is estimated that divorce rate in 2020 and 2021 will be higher than previous years in the U.S. and around the world.

In some countries men commit suicide due to the lack of income and losing their jobs and those who are in deep financial trouble. Many men run away from their homes in Japan either because they have lost their jobs or fall into financial difficulties. All these are due to the pandemic. The impact of the pandemic to individual has been the most difficult in 2020. These difficulties have been world-wide and the impact will continue even post-pandemic and a new deadly future virus may emerge more deadly than the Coronavirus.

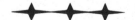

Impact on Society

The negative effect of the pandemic on society has been more damaging than ever. Uprising and riots in all 50 states in the United States and around the world in recent time (2020) reflects discriminations, burn outs, injustices and killings across the United States. Individual frustration because of the pandemic, lack of income, isolation combined with lost job, unemployment, financial hardship, social gathering regulations, lack of food have contributed to the uprising. The language of discrimination is being heard across the United States that has spread to all 50 states and cross the world, where there have been hundreds of arrests and curfews declared.

The society of the future will have to be more adaptive
with the change. Change in all sectors of the society. It is
a top-down process in making a change and it starts with
individuals. In reality, the chances of individual change
are somewhat limited. People will continue to do the same
activities as they have done in the past. So the notion of
starting each sector of the society with an unchangeable
blank slate will soon become obsolete and they go back
to the hardship. The challenge will be to devise and plan
streamlined processes slowly in order for the change to
occur gradually. One example is opening up the economy
and businesses while the pandemic is still affecting social
well-being.

Not only had the USA difficulties in controlling the
pandemic nationally but also controlling the discrimination
uprising at the same time. The public demonstration and

group gathering in masses in one place will have further spread the virus as much as 5 times higher than social distancing. Affected cases will overload hospitals and they would be unable to provide proper healthcare to infected people and non-Covid patients. The virus may have not been the direct cause of the uprising but has contributed to it. How? Restrict social regulations, economy pressure, isolation, unemployment, lack of income, lost jobs, discrimination, racism, lack of food and many other social issues that were fueled by the pandemic for the uprise.

Viruses have infected our society over years and limited our social activities, disturb our economy, broke family units and created recession in many countries. Viruses such as the SARS and the Covid-19 radically altered the very nature of global politics in just a few short months. Thousands of lives could have been saved if the control of the virus taken seriously by individuals who carried the virus and by government of nations that took the deadly virus light and not enforcing safety regulation on time to stop the pandemic.

Spawned variety of economic trends in respect to the growth that caused many sectors of the country to forget about the possibility of an attack by a killer virus such as "Coronavirus" that killed millions worldwide (CNN News), The effect of killer viruses as such will have profound consequences on current and the next generation globally. We have experienced both the benefits and perils of a truly global economy before the pandemic, with both Wall Street and Main Street feeling the pangs of economic dislocation half a world away. At the same time, we have fully entered into a new arena in the information age that may provide

a little help to prevent the spared of such viruses. Today, it
is almost impossible to imagine that the development of a
Coronavirus vaccine would be possible in a short time in
spite of new techno medical development. Lack of data and
transparency from Chinese government in respect to the
Coronavirus has delayed processes to move fast enough in
controlling the Virus. With stunning speed, the Coronavirus
has profoundly changed the way we live, work and socialize
and as a consequence, we have truly entered into a new down
fall economy and a new way of socializing phenomenal. We
never thought about social distancing or isolation before the
pandemic. This change virtually affected every individual,
family, social behavior and produced a pervasive demand for
continuous medical innovation to fight the virus and future
deadly viruses alike.

We have moved away from a prosperous economy to a bad economy that may take us years to overcome because of the Covid-19. 1 in 4 American workers have filed for unemployment benefits during the pandemic. This shift, in turn, places an unprecedented premium on financing the development of the vaccine for the Covid-19 and the discovering of the accelerated medical technology in finding a vaccine with the greatest speed. Another major medical trend has been the fragmentation for a drug approval process through FDA (Food & Drug Administration) in the USA. In order to bring about the development of medical equipment such as ventilators, gloves, gowns and other protective medical equipment, FDA approval process has not been fast enough to accommodate for the need.

There has been a growing appreciation that medical doctors, nurses, medical helpers and other similar groups of workers may have very different preferences in terms of helping the Covid-19 victims and how they want to assist the weak and the sick. According to Pew Research Center survey early in June 2020, they found 55% of these workers experiencing financial difficulties. Even prior to the pandemic, finances were a major source of problem for these groups of workers. As these healthcare workers continue to return to work every day, the healthcare leaders have to make them feel like they are being appreciated and make them comfortable voicing their concerns. In order to make life better for these healthcare workers and U.S. workers, major changes need to happen in many areas of the society.

If we refer to the theories of social behavior and review the historical data on the basis of social change we will see that theorists such as Toynbee (1957), Comte (1858) and Spencer (1988) have developed several ideas from which one can draw a picture of human nature and social change.

Depending from which extremes of the spectrum a person

selects his ideas; there could be broad social ramifications.

The purpose of changing the social behavior and the change

in social policies are to affect the knowledge, values, attitudes

and beliefs of the people within the society. The logical

outcome should be a change in social behavior. Historically

two basic lessons underscored by all change implementation

models reviewed here are: (a) the change process typically

occurs in multiple steps that take a considerable amount of

time and money to unfold, and efforts to bypass steps seldom

yield a satisfactory result, and (b) mistakes in any step can slow

implementation, as well as negate hard-won progress. Both

lessons are valuable for all those involved in understanding

and implementing the social change.

Despite of the pandemic all sectors of society starting with individuals, groups, organizations, and industries such as agricultural, retail, hospitality, manufacturing and service sectors and all level of government will need to do the process of change in order to make the society better. The first step is to plan for the change in order to define the processes needed for the change. The second step is to rethink the role of human beings in the society and the processes involved in making a social change. Redefining opportunities and responsibilities for millions of people in a society absent of mass formal employment is likely to be the single most pressing social issue after the pandemic arrival.

The steady upward climb in unemployment in the USA in each decade becomes even more troubling when organizations add the growing number of foreign workers replacing national U.S. workers who are in search of full-time employment and the number of discouraged workers who are no longer looking for a job because of the unfear competition with foreign workers. According to U.S. Bureau of Labor Statistics (2020), "in mid-2020 more than 50+ million people were unemployed. Many of the unemployed were so discouraged in finding a job that they stopped looking for a job all together. Peter Drucker (1993) notes that "the disappearance of domestic labor as a key factor of production is going to emerge as the critical unfinished business of capitalist society." (p. 12). According to President Trump that has repeatedly mentioned there will be overwhelming number of jobs available for everyone once the pandemic has disappeared. The fact that the Coronavirus is an unknown virus and there is a lot to learn from this killer virus, but this virus may never disappear.

Suppression of the pandemic can be preferred but needs to be maintained for as long as the virus is circulating in the human population or until a vaccine becomes available, otherwise the virus will quickly rebound when social measures are relaxed. Even if the measures are not relaxed the responsibility of prevention is on individuals to obey policies and avoid mass gathering and wearing masks to maintain a process in which the spread of the virus becomes minimal.

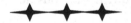

Social Change

Human beings are social creatures. Any social phenomenon is the result of a meaningful "interaction" between two or more individuals. It is through interaction that one may practice honesty or experience compassion. The fabric of social ecology is centered on human relationships, on feelings of intimacy, on companionship, fraternal bonds and stewardship. The qualities of individual interaction with others can easily be reduce to or replaced by fear. This fear can easily be created by number of known and unknown elements without the control of human being. One example of such a fear is a killer virus.

The effect of a pandemic on society could be tremendous and can change the core nature of the society and individual behavior. Coronavirus forced closure of businesses, restaurants, public locations; forced people to isolate and obey social distancing with restrict rules. The only entertainment was playing with smartphones and laptop computers and notebooks. Television and satellite dishes were heavily used in homes by family members to entertain themselves and socialize with others remotely while locked out. Social communications via social media overwhelmed the internet bandwidth. These social changes are more coherent in bigger metropolitan cities.

The Coronavirus had slow down and in some cases had stopped the social progress as occurred in every facet of the society, including the metaphysical, ethical, theological, intellectual and political realms. It created a social disorder and affected the core elements of the society. Aron (1968) writes, "Social disorders were rooted in the simultaneous existence of three incompatible philosophies: theological, metaphysical and positive" (p. 36). Lack of any of the named elements will create a social disorder.

One can see the social order could be created by the positive mind and the good behavior of the individual and their intellectual and moral progress toward benevolence among fellow humans. Another basic problem identified to cause social health issues is population growth. Population not necessary to more number of people but to density of population, the higher the concentration of human in a given space will create new wants and new problems such as the wide spread of a virus in a more populated cities like New Deli, Millan, Madrid and New York (May 2020). Viruses of any sort can quickly be spread among masses contaminating thousands of people. This occurred in India and China early when the pandemic started to spread. Population in many countries contributes to lawlessness, social chaos and sometimes creates social disorder. Lack of housing, for example, improper sewerage, shortage of food, lack of personal disciplines, lack of jobs and no income will usually cause problems in the society. Population growth generates new means of progress that might be hard to control and manage. If the population growth can somehow be controlled, we then would need to address how to better control the environment, climate and water and as a result better manage the spread of deadly viruses among masses. India and China both lack progress in this front. Their populations exceed to unmanageable proportion in recent years. Food shortages and famine will force populated countries to consume live animals. These practices of humans eating animals are still alive. It is a traditional practice in many parts of East Asian and China. Chinese diet include snakes, Chinese pangolin, live monkey brains, and bats, live fresh donkey, live baby duck embryos, baby mice, frogs, live birds and other wildlife. Due to religious reasons people in China forbidden to eat any portion of animals that are dead or cut to pieces, Animals must be alive for consumption (China Underground, 2020). Chinese were criticized for using wild animals for medicine, use as pets and for scientific research. Almost all wildlife animals are destined for restaurants and markets in Southern China. This is where the theory of bat-to-human infection (Coronavirus) came about.

The writer will examine the philosophy behind the social order and the social change in order to better understand the fabric of social behavior and elements of change to make a better society.

One of the knowledgeable theorists named Spencer (1969) proposed basis for distinguishing between types of societies and to differentiate between what he called **militant** and **industrial** societies. Spencer used this theory as his base for social organization through forms of social regulation. This classification is at variance with that based on stages of evolution.

Spencer (1851) writes, "The trait characterizing the **militant** structure throughout is that its units are coerced into their various combined actions. As the soldier's will is so suspended that he becomes in everything the agent of his officer's will, so is the will of the citizen in all transactions, private and public, overruled by that of the government. The cooperation by which the life of the militant society is maintained is compulsory cooperation ... just as in the individual organism the outer organs are completely subject to the chief nervous center" (pp. 19-23). The **industrial** type of society, in contrast, is based on voluntary cooperation and individual self-restrain.

One example, Spencer argues that "great civilizations can only arise in temperate zones...emerged out of the bloody throes of societal wars" (p. 178). Another great theorist named Toynbee (1961) mentioned adverse conditions cause civilizations to arise. Toynbee recognizes five different stimuli for a society to up rise; "hard countries, new ground, sudden military defeats, pressures and penalizations such as classes and races subjected to oppression, discrimination and exploitation" (p. 49). If we look at the linear developmental theories of many theorists in respect to social disorder and social uprising it becomes cloudier and more difficult to comprehend. Some believe that society guided itself in this progression and dismantlement and men had little influence over it.

All societies make change when change is inevitable, and rarely do they make changes when they are comfortable. Comte (1858) stated, "Man is a creature that must be stimulated or he will disintegrate" (p. 517). All civilizations seem to put forth their best efforts when challenged and to stagnate when times are good. It is only when there are strong injustices that the people will want change, and then only if they have been forced into it.

According to Spencer (1988) who builds a theory of social change, he writes "society is an organism". He uses his knowledge of biology to understand social phenomena. He believes that social change occurs as a result of physical, emotional and intellectual changes in individuals. The rate of the change is depended on the degree of the change in individual, some may become change agent and lead the change, others may force to change and often some individuals never want to change. But in general and in oppose to general belief, humans are capable of change either by force or voluntary, change for better or for worse. Social change includes cultural change, behavior change and change in one's mindset and attitude. Mindset definition refers to whether one believes qualities such as intelligence and talent are fixed or changeable traits. People with a fixed mindset believe that these qualities are inborn, fixed, and unchangeable. Other people have flexible and changeable mindset and can easily adapt to change. Once one's mindset changes, everything on the outside will change along with it. Sometimes members of a society are often confronted by customs that differ from those which they have learnt to accept. New customs and practices are more readily adopted if one's mindset is more flexible. Changes in culture are always super imposed on existing culture especially during cultural contact. Cultural change leads to chain reaction, whenever a change is incorporated into the culture and becomes a social

necessity, new needs emerge, generating the desire for further

changes to complement or supplement the original change.

One cannot manage change; one can only be a head of

the change (Drucker, 1999). Change has become an inherent

part of our life before and during the pandemic. What is more

significant is the rapid accelerating velocity of change for

worse rather than change for better. The rapidly increasing

velocity of change during the pandemic warps individuals'

time and space, bending the very shape of the economy

globally. It is not just simply a matter of doing the same things

to make a change but the change should be by doing things

different and for better and it should happen faster for ever

changing events. The massive demands for change imposed by

time compression has forced some individuals to compete the

change cycle and innovate simultaneously in multiple venues

in overlapping time frames and finding creative ways to design and implement the change in different ways in society to cope with the hardship created by Covid-19.

Spencer (1874) writes, "Social change occurs as a result of individual's change, therefore, is limited by the rate at which individual changes and pass on those individual modifications to succeeding generations" (pp. 401-404). Social change, in essence, creates new needs; new needs require new ideas which in turn require changes in the physical, emotional and intellectual traits of individuals.

Spencer (1874) writes, "Society is an aggregate of individuals and change in society could take place only when the individual members of that society had changed and developed (pp. 366-367). Individuals are, therefore, "primary", individual development was "egoistic" and associations with others largely instrumental and contractual. As the writer previously mentioned, to make a change one needs to be motivated to make the change. Individual efforts in a group will create a sense of need to make a change as a group. Group efforts to make the change will cause the social to change. It is a top down process that starts with individuals and ends at the social level (Exhibit A).

Public education is truly the key element in initiating the social change process. Human are capable of change, the question is to what extend the public wants to change? Do we need to force the change? Does the education necessary for individual or for the society to change? Do we need general public education? It seems, however, if education intends to become an agent change and constructive, transformative of change, some sort of evolving social consciousness should permeate the aim and content of education.

The change process begins with the "individual" as the fundamental unit of social change. Next is a social interaction. Any social phenomenon is the result of a meaningful "interaction" between two or more individuals. Comte (1974) writes, "A social state is both a continuous state of individual satisfaction ... also a continuous state of sacrifice" (p. 236). Interaction is necessary not only for material survival, but also for the emergence of meanings and values that comprises the non-material aspects of human life. If this interaction is taken away by means of isolation because of a pandemic, for example, the individual satisfaction will not meet the demand for wellbeing and the change will not happen because of it.

A quick change to the social development efforts fall short of their objectives because most important step is not taken or is conducted superficially and the changes are subject to resistance and elimination. Resistance to change is a process of conscious or unconscious blocking as a means to seeking safety. It is believed that to overcome the resistance one makes the individual or a society uncomfortable enough with the old way that they would try to find something new. If the change is not successful in implementing for an individual or for a society, conflict will occur when there is a gap or disparity between the social levels and more often disparity and conflict occurs between member of a society and their government.

One of the challenges for top political leaders will be to determine when, how and in what situations they can amend new legislations for social change, safeguard the society, reform policies and legal processes in order to eliminate injustices and discrimination of any forms in the USA and in any other country. Every nation in the globe must rethink the role of human beings in their society and the processes involved in making a better society by changing the culture over time and changing the processes in proper time. The strategic imperatives described will create a compelling need for some new and unconventional social change.

Social Disorder

The history of humankind is one of continuing cycles of birth, growth, breakdown and disintegration of civilizations. The whole process as being intimately tied up with the functioning of elite and their relationships with the masses, both the internal and external proletariats. Historically no civilization continues to grow indefinitely and there is a breakdown, which occurs when the creative elite and top tier of the society no longer functions adequately, the majority no longer gives its allegiance to and imitates the elite and social unity disintegrates, one good example of this is the Trump administration and how the Whitehouse (elite) disintegrating components of the society in all levels in the time of pandemic. Society continues as an identifiable civilization but it is stagnant as far as cultural behavior is concerned. Like an individual who has lost virtually everything but the capacity to breathe and eat and cling to life and lingered on but contributed nothing to the social values.

History has been repeating itself. There have been many forms of protests in the USA for many reasons. Like protests for the 15th Amendment in 1870, protests for women Liberation in 1960, protests for jobs & freedom in 1963, protests for the civil rights act of 1965, protests for anti-Vietnam war in 1969, protests for solidarity day in 1981, protests for anti-nuclear in 1982, protests for Iraq war in 2003, and now the George Floyd protests in 2020. In the U.S. political protests have a rich past, with varied degrees of success in accomplishing what they originally set out to do. Protests in other countries are not so successful. In some countries thousands of people die in protects and they are not as lucky as people in the U.S.A to get results through protects.

Racial discrimination is as pressing and reoccurring as most recent days (25 May, 2020) like the killing of George Floyd of Minneapolis and similar killings across the USA in recent months and years which was and still is a primary cause of the breakdown of society and the uprising. This has caused a major disintegration of civilizations at the time of happening and possibly continues to the future. Discrimination is not an easy problem to solve and will only grow worse as more African-American being killed by brutality of law enforcement officers and neighborhood police. According to Pascoe (2009) racial discrimination is any discrimination against individuals on the basis of their skin color, or racial or ethnic origin. Individuals can discriminate by refusing to do business with, socialize with, or share resources with people of a certain group. Governments can discriminate in a de facto fashion or explicitly in law, for example through policies of racial segregation, disparate enforcement of laws, or disproportionate allocation of resources. Some jurisdictions in the USA have anti discrimination laws which prohibit the government or individuals from discriminating based on race and sometimes other factors in various circumstances. Some institutions and laws use affirmative action to attempt to overcome or compensate for the effects of racial discrimination. In some cases, this is simply enhanced recruitment of members of underrepresented groups; in other cases, there are firm racial quotas. Opponents of strong remedies like quotas characterize them as reverse discrimination, where members of a dominant or majority group are discriminated against.

The common American notion is that most American are geographically from Europe with European background and have European ancestry of light skin so called "White", and other European immigrants like Irish Americans and

Italian Americans whose whiteness was challenged faced legal discrimination. American laws has divided the population into 5 races; White, American Indian and Alaska Native, Asian, Black or African American, Native Hawaiian. South African (white minorities) laws which divided the population into certain classifications; whites from Europe and blacks from Africa sub-Saharan and that often caused problems of interpretation when dealing with people from other areas, such as the rest of the Mediterranean Basin, Asia, North Africa usually resulting in lower level of living and causing legal discrimination. Discrimination based on skin color, is closely related to racial discrimination, as skin color is often used as a proxy for race in everyday interactions, and is one factor used by legal systems that apply detailed criteria.

It is imperative that private firms, business associations, communities, and intermediary organizations address complex problems of discrimination in the basis of race, sex, religious, age and national origin. Discrimination is the act of making distinctions between human beings based on the groups, classes, or other categories to which they are perceived to belong. People may discriminate on the basis of age, caste, criminal record, height, weight, physical appearance, disability, family status, gender identity, gender expression, generation, genetic characteristics, marital status, nationality, color, race and ethnicity, religion, sex and sex characteristics, sexual orientation, political ideology, social class, personality, species, as well as other categories. According to Wikipedia (2020), discrimination occurs when individuals or groups are treated unfairly in a way which is worse than the way people are usually treated.

Discrimination can cause chronic stress lead to a wide variety of physical and mental health problems. Indeed, perceived discrimination has been linked to issues including anger, anxiety, depression, obesity, high blood pressure and substance abuse and sometimes death and suicide (Pascoe, 2009). Some define the discrimination as the unfair or prejudicial treatment of people and groups based on characteristics such as race, gender, age or sexual orientation. The most important question is: Can discrimination be eliminated? It can be eliminated, once everyone starts treating all people equally. It starts with the government and public education and enforcement. Treading all people equally is not easy for many people as their core belief has been set to separate themselves from others as a superior group. That can be seen in many countries as we speak. The discrimination might be resolved to some extent if government initiates the process of anti-discrimination education for masses. It is a top-down process, from the Whitehouse to federal government and down to states and to each city in states. Adapting the change in all sectors of the government should include top level of government officials from Supreme Court to justice department to law enforcements to public and private organizations and to individuals. This will have a domino effect in changing the society behavior toward discrimination. If we can only focus in one category of discrimination like the "race" and to eliminate the race discrimination or even minimize it we will learn how to deal with minimizing and removing discrimination as a whole in all other categories of discrimination such as sex, age, gender, religion, disability, national origin, pregnancy, equal pay and others.

Another problem is the class conflict and color classification set by the U.S. government years ago. There are 3 major racial groups that can be defined in many countries; 1) white, 2) black and 3) other multi-racial minorities. The United States has a racially and ethnically diverse population.

At the federal level, race and ethnicity have been categorized separately. As of July 2019 African American was the 2nd largest racial minority of 13% in the U.S. Hispanic and Latino American counted for 18% of the population, Asian 6%, Native American (Alaska, Hawaii, Pacific Islanders) 1.3%, the White, non-Hispanic population made up of 60% of the U.S. total population (2016). These numbers have increased by certain extend in 2020 to reflect the actual total U.S. population of 331+ million (World-o-Meter, 2020).

From the total U.S. population of 331+ million 10% of this number is wealthy and rich. The middle class bear the burden of paying more taxes and they are referred to as pay-check to pay-check groups. The under privileged group are minorities and those who live under poverty line. This group is more vulnerable catching the pandemic in greater number. They are referred to as the bottom of the barrel in the society. Some individuals in this group will always be ready to take advantage of bad situation in creating social disorder and riots. So sort of revenge against other groups and even their own government. Among this group many don't have anything to lose.

One other known group is the ANTIFA (Anti-Fascist Political Activist) movement in the United States that is a militant, left-wing, anti-fascist political activist movement which comprises autonomous activist groups that aim to achieve their political objectives through the use of "direct action" rather than through policy reform. Activists engage in variety of protests and tactical movements to achieve their goals including digital activism, property damage, physical violence and harassment against those whom they identify as fascist, racist or on the far-right (The New York Times, 2020).

Individuals involved in this movement tend to hold anti-capitalist views and subscribe to a range of ideologies such as anarchism, socialism, communism, liberalism and social democracy. President Donald Trump refers to this group as "Terrorist". This group rose When Italian dictator Benito Mussolini consolidated power under his National Fascist Party in the mid-1920s, an oppositional anti-fascist movement surfaced both in Italy and countries such as the United States. Many anti-fascist leaders in the United States were syndicalist, anarchist, and socialist émigrés from Italy with experience in labor organizing and militancy (Tavernise, 2020). Ideologically, Antifa in America sees itself as the successor to anti-Nazi activists of the 1930s; European activist groups that originally organized to oppose World War II era fascist dictatorships re-emerged in the 1970s and 1980s to oppose white supremacy and skinheads and eventually spread to America. After World War II, but prior to the development of the modern Antifa movement, violent confrontations with fascist elements continued sporadically (Kuo, 2020).

Modern Antifa politics can be traced to opposition to the infiltration of Britain's punk scene by white power skinheads in the 1970s and 1980s and the emergence of neo-Nazism in Germany following the fall of the Berlin Wall (Clamp, 2020). In Germany, young leftists, including anarchists and punk fans, renewed the practice of street-level anti-fascism. Columnist Peter Beinart (2012) writes "in the late '80s, left-wing punk fans in the United States began following suit, though they initially called their groups Anti-Racist Action (ARA) on the theory that Americans would be more familiar with fighting racism than they would be with fighting fascism.". Antifa group in the U.S. amid to make the racism go away and make a change for better by the means of disruption and chaos and force the government to adapt to new policies.

What is clear is that the society of the future will need to adapt to a new behavior and work together in making the

social change for better society and to succeed and become
one unit less dependent on the independent actions of
disaggregated individuals and racism. To succeed, society in
addition to the government will have to develop a competency
in the design of new policies to eliminate racial discrimination
as the Covid-19 pandemic or any future viruses should not
overshadow the processes.

Regardless of social belongingness like ARA, Antifa,
Black Lives Matter, or any other groups, discrimination in
any forms or any shapes should not be tolerated. We need
to work together to raise awareness of discrimination against
African Americans or any other groups of minorities. New
policies should be set to eliminate discrimination of all kinds.
Employment hiring should not be based on race, or sex,
sexual preference, religion, origin and age. Social behavior
should not create the impression that one race or sex is either

stronger and better or weaker than the others, which leads

to resentment of the excluded race, when qualification-based

hiring practices should be the only consideration (Debate.

org, 2020). As recently as 30 years ago, classified ads for

employment were divided, men wanted in one section and

women wanted in another. It was unusual to see women or

minorities as television news anchors and there were far fewer

woman and minorities in jobs as supervisors, firefighters,

police officers doctors and college professors. "Since the

passage of the Civil Rights Act of 1964, minorities and

woman have made real economic progress. Their wages and

employment rates increased." (Herman, 1999, p. 209). Women

are far more able to contribute to their families' incomes, and

have become a major force in business and political life.

"Hispanics and newer immigrant populations are

emerging as strong contributors to the U.S. economy."

(Herman, 1999, p. 2009). A generation of professional's minorities and African American provide role models for young and minority youths.

According to U.S. Equal Employment Opportunity Commission (EEOC), "there have been 12,500 claims of discrimination filed with the agency based on race, color, national origin, gender, religion, age, or disability were found to be meritorious allegations or were resolved in favor of the complaining party. It is also interesting to know that "it is not possible to know how many cases of the same are not documented and are not known, such as discrimination based on sexual orientation, have not been remedied because current law does not reach them." (Report, 2020).

The black middle class has been growing in recent years but discrimination in African-American employment hiring is and has been a continuing problem. This has been demonstrated by audit studies in which white and minority or male and female job seekers are given similar resumes and sent to the same firms to apply for the same job. These studies often find that employers are less likely to interview or offer a job to an African-American or minority application. For that matter many African Americans or other minorities left behind the America mainstream unless the policies from the top force to change in order to eliminate the discrimination.

According to ABC News on June 15, 2020 "The U.S. Supreme Court historically ruled that employment discrimination on the basis of sexual orientation or gender identity to be prohibited under the civil rights law". A major victory for the Civil Rights Act of 1964, which makes it illegal for employers to discriminate because of a person's sex among other factors. More of the same change should happen in the U.S. to make life better for the minorities and those of color.

In spite of the Civil Rights Act of 1964 the Killing of George Floyd in Minneapolis (May 25, 2020) sparked fury over racism and police brutality. That prompted President Trump to take his first concrete steps less than a month later on June 16, 2020 to address growing national outcry over police brutality that killed George Floyd, Even as he offered a staunch defense of law enforcement that left little question about his allegiances. President Trump announced an executive order that among other steps to create a federal database of police officers with a history of using excessive force. He mentioned "the problem rested on a small number of individual officers, it is a very small percentage but nobody wants to get rid of them more than the really good and great police officers" (Saul Loeb/AFP, 2020).

It seems that any changes to social order will overwhelm our ability to cope emotionally and make our society unable to manage our affairs in planning for our future. The impact of past viruses and the change on society in the past centuries was relatively isolated and cyclic, but now as society grows and evolve; they are continuously subjected to more similar deadly virus attack and biological warfare. At the same time society is also subject to the influence of internal and external factors that may lead to chaos and disruption of the progress in the society. According to Webster's dictionary (1988), the meaning of change is "to transform, alter, to convert" (p. 234). Our world now seems defined more by chaos and sudden changes for worse than by stability and fairness.

Once a change has been accepted and implemented by a society, the initiators of the change (in this case the government or groups) must keep working with the members and emphasizing the positive effects of the change, otherwise, the society may slowly lapse into its old habits. Lewin (1935) states, "The direction of the field force plays an important part in such intelligent behavior as it has to do with detour problems" (p. 82).

A critical social issue in change and managing change is dealing effectively with the emotions in individual affairs. Kubler-Ross (1969) is one of the most important contributors to our understanding of the human response to stress and resistance to change. Kubler-Ross (1969) identifies five stages of human response to dramatic change: "1) denial and isolation, 2) anger, 3) bargaining, 4) depression and resignation and 5) acceptance" (p. 41). According to Kubler-Ross (1969), "Denial is an outgrowth of the failure of most individuals to anticipate and thus begin to emotionally prepare for traumatic events in their lives" (p. 41-43).

For most people, the idea of "it could never happen to me" all too quickly transforms into "it hasn't happened to me", when disaster actually occurs it transforms to "why it happened to me". Kubler-Ross (1969) writes, "Denial is usually accompanied by isolation from any part of the environment, which may tend to remind the individual that the traumatic change has in fact occurred" (p. 342). Denial and isolation are emotional protection for the individual and thus are often not principled or thoughtful opposition to the change, though they are often mistaken for being so. Kubler-Ross (1969) notes that, this response "is analogous to the phenomenon of psychological flight, which is the tendency of individuals to flee danger" (p. 343). The alternative phenomenon, psychological flight, is analogous to the next Kubler-Ross stage. Kubler-Ross (1969) explains, "Anger is a familiar but often misinterpreted response to traumatic change ... as the veil of denial falls from the eyes of the individual, and the pain of the change begins to be felt, anger is an inevitable result" (p. 42).

Feelings of unfair treatment, race discrimination, resentment about past injustices and police brutality and killings create an infinite array of other injustice actions serve to fuel one's anger. As we have seen this kind of anger after the killing of George Floyd in Minneapolis Minnesota in May of 2020 in the USA. Kubler-Ross writes, "In contrast to the stage of denial, the stage of anger is very difficult to cope with from the point of view of individuals and family. The reason is that anger displaced in all directions and projected on to the environment at times almost at random" (p. 64).

Additionally, groups of people with such fears often find comfort in sharing their fears with one other, creating a social fear, chaos and looting thus making the change process more difficult. Kubler-Ross (1983) writes, "Fears are gifts to us since they preserve life ... either knowingly or unconsciously, we pass our acquired fears along to our children and are not aware until it is too late that these cause indescribable damage and pain" (p. 61).

According to Kubler-Ross (1969), "when denial and anger fail, the change disappear, the next resistance to change is bargaining" (p. 64). This period is an effort by the individual, in every way possible, to mitigate the impact of the change and to buy time. Individuals may accept parts of the change phenomenon and deny others. In this stage, the individual wants to make a deal between the change factors that seem to be inevitable and those that do not.

"Depression is the final barrier for accepting the change" (Kubler-Ross, 1969, p. 342). It may start with reaction or depression over what has been occurred or lost. Then it is anticipatory depression over what is expected to be lost. Resignation usually follows. In this stage rational action on the part of the individual or a society usually begins.

"Acceptance is not necessarily either happy or satisfied or unhappy and dissatisfied ... what it is clear is the individual finally sees the truth and is dealing with it, effectively or not, as a reality" (Kubler-Ross, 1969, p. 43).

While more must be done in the area of discrimination, any new discrimination resolutions should signify an important step toward greater engagement between local, state, and federal elected officials and African American and any other minorities to end harmful stereotyping and discrimination. There is a lot that the White House and the U.S. government can do to eliminate the discrimination of any sort in the USA. Discrimination has no place in the U.S. or anywhere else in the world for that matter and does not speak to the values of any great societies. We all should pledge to work with our political leaders and congress to change the policies and to end senseless violence, racism and injustice.

Change and reform to justice and police brutality should be at
the top of the list for policy makers.

Social change and policy change will occur regardless of
the social reaction and oppositions. But to what extend the
change will affect the society is yet to be seen. The evidence
is clear that discrimination and exclusion persist in our society
today everywhere and is not limited to the U.S. but it exists
globally. From persecution of Muslims in Myanmar to Hafez
al-Assad Hama massacre in February 1982 killing thousands
and displacing millions Syrians, to many years of conflict
between Palestinians and Israeli occupying Palestinians
territories and discriminations, to Hong Kong conflict with
mainland China undermining Hong Kong's autonomy and
infringing civil liberties, to Zimbabwe where there has
been increasing racism against the white farmers in Africa,
to Malaysia enforced discriminatory laws limiting access to

university education for Chinese students who are citizens by birth of Malaysia, and many other laws explicitly favoring Malays remain in force and finally after the September 11, 2001, there has additionally been an outpouring of violent racial hatred by a minority of people in Western countries against people that look Middle Eastern. Since the horrific terrorist attacks on the United States on September 11, 2001, Security concerns have understandably increased the same goes for racial profiling and discrimination. Australia has had a very racist past in which apartheid has been practiced and where indigenous Aboriginal people have lost almost all their land and suffered many prejudices. Greece has one of the worst records in the European Union for racism against ethnic minorities, according to the BBC (2020). Anti-immigrant sentiment has long been high, especially against ethnic Albanians, who form the largest minority. The grant finale of all was the Adolph Hitler killing million Jews and dislocating millions of Europeans. Hitler blamed the Jews for everything that was wrong with the world. He believed that Germany was weak and in decline due to the 'Jewish influence'. Hitler divided the world population into high and low races. The Germans belonged to the high race nation and Jews to the low race. He also had specific notions about other peoples. During the 1930s, he did everything he could to expel the Jews from German society. Once the war had started, the Nazis resorted to mass murder. Nearly six million Jews were murdered during the Holocaust and around two-thirds of them were Europe's Jewish population.

Impact on Economy

We are rapidly shifting from a good economy to a disastrous economy in a very short time since the great deprecation. The economic impacts of the Covid-10 pandemic have been far and wide, hurting virtually every industry and leaving tens of millions of people without paychecks to pay their bills. The negative effect of the pandemic on economy has been more damaging than ever before. Unemployment, financial hardship, social gathering restrictions, lack of food and home isolation has contributed to the uprising in recent weeks in many countries (May 2020). Not only had we had to control the pandemic across nations and minimize the spread of virus but also nationally controlling the up-rise and demonstrations in protest of racial discrimination. The

Coronavirus may have not been in direct cause of the social disturbance in recent weeks and months but it has contributed to it in a great deal.

Startling breakthroughs in information technology have irreversibly altered the ability to conduct medical research in finding a cure and that may be due to business innovation and ability to spend multi million dollars in R&D in medical field. The cause of slow process in finding a cure for the Coronavirus pandemic are that businesses constrained by the limitations of time, space and economy in addition to difficulties in medical procedures and FDA approval. Economists have been using the SARS pandemic to put the Coronavirus outbreak in context. The 2003 SARS pandemic was estimated to have shaved between 0.5% and 1% off of China's growth that year and cost the global economy about $40 billion (or 0.1% of global Gross Domestic Product (GDP).

The Covid-19 pandemic, which like SARS originated in China, differs in a few key ways. China's economy accounted for roughly 4% of the world's GDP in 2003; it now commands 16.3%, which is 4 times as much in 2020. If the Coronavirus has a similar effect on China as SARS, the impact on global growth would have been worse.

According to China News (2020) China's growth is weaker than it was in 2003 after years of rapid economic development, China's growth stands at 6%, the lowest it has been since 1990. Its confidence had been shaken by the dual effects of general economic deceleration and the U.S.-China trade war escalation and now the spread of the recent pandemic weaken the China's economy. As the world is in the middle of the battle against the pandemic, two class actions were filed against China for "damages suffered as the result of the Coronavirus pandemic" before the U.S. District Court in Florida and Texas, shocking the Chinese legal community (News.cgtn.com/news, 2020).

The American plaintiffs in these lawsuits alleged that the Chinese authorities knew that the Covid-19 was dangerous and capable of causing a pandemic and yet they slowly responded to the novel Coronavirus by "proverbially putting their head in the sand," sparking the global pandemic outbreak. They even go as far as alleging that the Covid-19 virus escaped from the Wuhan Institute of Virology, which they claimed was a Biological Weapons Research Lab run by the Chinese government. Therefore, they demand that Chinese authorities should pay damages to all American victims for their economic and non-economic damages, injury and loss related to the outbreak of the Covid-19, an award in excess of 20 trillion U.S. dollars (Views of CGTN, 2020). Many European countries are also in pursuing of the same. At the same time countries like India, Germany, Australia and Nigeria have blamed China for failing to take precautionary measures to stop the virus spreading globally (CNBC, 2020).

The Coronavirus spreads more quickly than SARS but so far seems Covid-19 to have much higher mortality rate. For its part, China did not respond more quickly to the Coronavirus outbreak than it did with SARS, employing unprecedented confinement measures in some areas for SARS and later for the Coronavirus in Wuhan. But the Chinese measures were not good enough to contain the virus on time and either purposely or otherwise spread the virus all over the world. These Chinese measures, while prudent, have created long-term economic pain for all nations of the world and caused major headaches for the supply-and-demand side. Families, companies, and governments are deeper in debt now than they were when SARS hit. What was the reason(s) for the Chines to take such a wrong action against the world? We shall never find out but we can guess may be Chinese wanted to bring the world economy down or may be to change the mode of the U.S. 2020 election? Whatever the reasons, the new weapon of warfare is going to be the biological war in the future.

Deutsche Bank (2020) released analysis showing the world's major economies harboring the highest debt levels of the past 150 years, with World War II as an exception. They all still need to continue repaying that debt. Jobs, customers, consumers and tax revenues decline are weakening economy because of the pandemic. These costs will leave less money to spend on other things such as development of a deadly virus vaccine by many countries under the debt. According to Garrett Parker (2020), top 10 countries that are under the debt with Japan with its population of 127,185,332 has the highest national debt in the world at 234.18% of its GDP ($9.087

trillion USD), followed by Greece at 181.78% ($379 billion USD) as the 2nd highest country under the debt. Portugal at $264 billion (ranked 3), Italy at $2.48 trillion (ranked 4), Bhutan at $2.33 billion (ranked 5), Cyprus at $21.64 billion (ranked 6), Belgium at $456.18 billion (ranked 7), United States of America at $19.23 trillion (ranked 8), Spain at $1.24 trillion (ranked 9) and Singapore at $254 billion (ranked 10). These numbers are growing by days due to the pandemic. Germany has the strongest economy in the Europe. Large amounts of debt often exacerbate an economic slowdown, especially if central banks can do little to ease that burden by cutting interest rates.

The world looks different financially now than the last global virus outbreak in 2003. Global growth is already slow and financial markets already have very low interest rate which means that central banks in almost every major country have little ammunition with which to mitigate any potential economic fallout. This puts greater pressure on governments of the nations to use the power of their purse to counter the economic fallout from this pandemic. The current situation will create lots of uncertainty over the longer term. The global economy downfall due to the killer virus is a new way of global financial warfare. Any nuclear attack would have killed many and damage one city or two, but a killer virus like the Covid-19 and future deadly viruses alike will kill as many as multiple nuclear attacks in multiple countries and ruin the global economy in matter of weeks.

Disruptions to global supply chains are one of the clearest effects of the pandemic. Looking more closely at global supply chains, there have already been significant disruptions with the list of manufacturers forced to decrease production or cut jobs in their plants. Germany cutting thousands of jobs in its auto manufacturing sector, Japan the same, England the same, Saudi Arabia cutting jobs in many oil and refinery productions and the same goes for all other international manufacturing organizations. Not to mention that many industries in the U.S. cutting jobs by thousands. For example American Airlines cut 19,000 jobs, AT&T cut 37,000 jobs, MGM Resorts International 18,000 jobs, Coca-Cola Company 4,000 jobs, Boeing 19,000 jobs, Raytheon Technologies Corp 8,000 jobs, Salesforce.com Inc. 1,000 jobs, Estee Lauder Cosmetics 2,000 jobs and Bed Bath & beyond Inc. 2, 800 jobs.

It is possible that many workers around the world may not be able or not willing to show up to work because of the threat of the Coronavirus or habit of getting used to staying home longer than normal and getting used to not going to work. This will further slowdown the economy recovery. These challenges affect not just traditional industries such as retail, entertainments, hospitality and many others but also increasingly affecting high-tech industries such as smart phones and computer manufacturing. As a consequence of these supply chain disruptions, firms cannot finish their own production and thus cannot bring their products to market globally. The result is reduced economic recovery and growth. One example is Apple Corporation. The holdup for 5G iPhones comes as the pandemic has weakened global consumer demand and thrown a wrench into manufacturing operations across Asia, according to the Wall Street Journal. (New York Post, 2020).

The virus will not only affect supply, but some sectors of the economy may also experience decline in demand and big reductions in revenue because of the overall effects of the pandemic on the global economy. There are two separate effects to consider. One effect is that people will buy less of some goods and services because they are afraid of potential exposure to the virus. As many people feel increasingly uneasy about the spread of the virus in their country, it is foreseeable that they will further cut back on some goods and services and that possibly causes a decrease on their emergency savings. The second effect is when firms are forced to close by new restrictions, workers likely will receive less money than they otherwise would have expected and in some instances will receive no pay. As a result, these workers will have less to spend, again cutting overall demand. A fall in demand that follows a supply shock constitutes a one-two punch that will further impact economic activities, although the size of these affects will largely be in longer term rather than a quick fix.

As such effects proliferate around the world; many global exporters will find it harder to sell their goods and products around the globe, which will have negative repercussions for global economy growth and further elimination of jobs in many counties. This new trouble phenomenon will most likely continue to last for years to come.

Political polarization and conflicting policies on regulation combined with the pandemic have led to people and firms thinking twice before investing or expanding. The chart below indicates the global economic before and after Coronavirus that has increased over the past few years with a spike in 2020 that caused the Coronavirus to begin spreading globally.

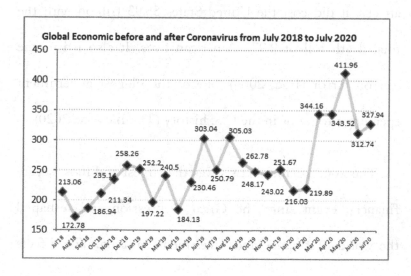

In addition to the already high level of U.S. foreign and international policy uncertainty, the effects of the pandemic outbreak have a commonality with the 9/11 in 2001 and financial crisis in 2008 and its unknown magnitude.

The 9/11 attacks had both immediate and long-term economic impacts, some of which continue to this day. The attacks caused the Dow to drop almost 700 points and deepened the 2001 recession. While it cost al-Qaeda an estimated $400,000-$500,000 to plan and carry out the attacks, it did cost the United States $5.93 trillion with the total death toll of 2,977 American lives. It also led to the war on terror (Iraq, 2003), one of the biggest government spending programs in the U.S. history (The Balance, 2020).

The 2008 financial crisis was the largest and most severe financial event since the Great Depression and reshaped the world of finance and investment banking. The effects are still being felt today, yet many people did not and still do not actually understand the causes or what took place. The underlying cause of the financial crisis in 2008 was a combination of debt and mortgage-backed assets. Since the end of WW2, house prices in the United States have been steadily rising. There have been a few financial fluctuations in between, but the trend has been upward causing a housing bubble. In the 1980s financial institutions and traders realized that the U.S. mortgages were an untapped asset and started to abuse the system by tapping to these assets that caused the values of securities that were tied to U.S. real estate to plummet, at the same time the Lehman Brothers filed for Chapter 11 bankruptcy protection on September 15, 2008 that remains the largest bankruptcy filing in U.S. history, holding over US$600 billion in assets causing a total chaos for the U.S. financial institutions and the world and that is known as the Global Financial Crisis (GFC).

The financial impact of the Covid-19 pandemic to the U.S. has been as bad as 9/11 and 2008 crisis, even worse with tremendous human life losses. To analyze the impact of the pandemic on the U.S. economy one can look at the state of Connecticut. According to Joe Courtney, the congressman of Connecticut, preliminary projections were that the Covid-19 pandemic will cost Connecticut cities and towns over $407 million in revenue, plus another $63 million in added costs as the Connecticut state begins to recover. Sum of $470 million lost for one small state. More or less the same goes for all other U.S. states. The pandemic has taken a huge chunk out of many U.S. states budget and their municipalities' piggy banks, leaving thousands of towns scrambling for cash and raising the prospect of major property tax hikes in addition to other drastic measures to regain the revenue lost due to the pandemic. According to Connecticut Mirror (News, 2020) local community leaders in the U.S. have been warned since mid-March of 2020 that the public health crisis, coupled with

the associated businesses and school shutdowns and massive

unemployment, would leave the U.S. finances in shambles.

To gain the lost revenue for the U.S. states some

drastic measures should be implemented such as reducing

state budgets by reducing the budget for law enforcement

department, fire department, healthcare organizations, higher

fees for public transportations, higher fees for highway use,

school budget reduction, doubling the state sales tax and

property taxes in addition to other similar measures.

There are uncertainties about the scale of the pandemic

on the U.S. economy, contagion rate, mortality rates,

risk of incidence and more. On top of all the usual online

misinformation and swirl of Conspiracy Theories, there are

questions about the accuracy of the health statistics coming

from China; number of deaths, number of cases, number of

recovered, virus transferred from animal-to-human theory and many other theories alike. The issue of credibility has only become more challenging during this crisis and it makes assessing the impact of the virus on the global economy that much more difficult. For many countries the effect of a killer pandemic such as the Covid-19 on economy will take more than ten (10) years to recover and for the 3rd world countries they may never recover.

Businesses are not the only ones that could pull back amid uncertainty. Families worried about contracting the virus that could cut spending on some items such as traveling and entertainments and going out dinning. Moreover, this health risk poses a real economic risk, as many households have inadequate health insurance, which could leave them with large hospital bills when they get sick, especially in the United

States with a very high cost of healthcare many individuals will go bankrupt because of it.

Banks and other financial institutions may restrict and reprice financial credit because they cannot properly assess short-term risks to particular borrowers, sectors, or countries. Less credit availability could make it harder for businesses, especially smaller ones to invest and grow. In the United States with a mass real estate mortgage loans many potential home buyers or first time buyers will find it harder to get a home loan or not being able to pay for the existing home mortgages and loans. Credit market uncertainty could then exacerbate the demand fallout from the pandemic. On economy wide scale, though, this means less spending and thus less growth, this will apply to first world countries like the USA, Germany, Sweden, New Zealand, Ireland, Canada, Netherlands, Australia, Norway and other European countries. Economy growth in 2nd world counties will stay low or none for some.

Countries such as Armenia, Bulgaria, Czech Republic, Hungary, Poland, Romania, Slovenia, Turkmenistan and Uzbekistan are in this category. In 3rd world counties mostly in the Middle East and Africa their economy will not growth at all and will even worsen and the financial hardship will remain for generations to come. Countries like Venezuela, Iran, Cuba, Sudan, North Korea, Libya, Ivory Coast, Congo and Zimbabwe may be considered as such. Other countries that are under the U.S.A trade or financial sanctions either unilaterally or in part include the Balkans, Belarus, Burundi, Central African Republic, Cuba, Democratic Republic of Congo, Hong Kong, Iran, Iraq, Lebanon, Libya, Mali, Nicaragua, North Korea, Somalia, Sudan, South Sudan, Syria, Ukraine/Russia, Venezuela, Yemen, and Zimbabwe. These countries may not recover from the pandemic financial hardship unless there is a change in government and/or the society.

There is also an international wrinkle to growing uncertainty. International financial investors could become worried about the unknown risks to the global economy because of the pandemic and future similar deadly viruses. They could look for the comfort of a safe investment. Traditionally, U.S. treasuries are seen as very safe investment. However, because of the pandemic, less money will be coming into the United States from abroad and that typically weakens the U.S. dollar and a weaker U.S. dollar will eventually make the U.S. economy weaker and that makes it more difficult for the U.S. firms to compete globally. It is very much like a domino effect; one will affect the other to fall.

Supply chain disruptions and the demand reduction and global economic uncertainty all happened against the backdrop of many firms and households straining under large amounts of debt, all because of the Covid-19 pandemic.

These debts have to be repaid even if the economy continues to recover in a slow paste and even if the pandemic has long gone. These debt services then leave less money for businesses and households to spend when their incomes drop. High debt levels will exacerbate the economic fallout from the pandemic for years to recover.

Prices on bonds with a range of maturities reflect an increasing possibility of a recession. Inversions are typically taken as a sign that financial markets worry about the longer-term outlook for the economy. Financial markets will see a growing risk of a recession because of economy hardship due to the pandemic. In the same vein, lower long-term interest rates mean that financial markets expect the USA Fed to cut interest rates further down (3.35% in June 2020), to reduce the risk of a recession (Top10.com, 2020). Many countries offer stimulus programs in the means of cash to families and businesses to boost the economy. Countries like China, Japan, Germany, India, UK, France, Italy, Brazil, Canada, Russia, S. Korea and Australia provided stimulus and financial relief to their people. The United States had disbursed largest rescue package of $2.5 trillion in cash to families. This amount is by far greater stimulus than any country. This program increased federal debt by only about 9% (April 2020). The USA already had $23 trillion in debt before the pandemic but need to pay off or write-off this debt someday (The Guardian, 2020).

Potentially massive externalities related to the pandemic alter conventional economic thinking. The spread of the Covid-19 pandemic has begun to affect financial markets, but it is uncertain how severely the pandemic will strain the broader financial system globally in moving forward. As global financial markets become more volatile and more economically vulnerable, global economy will suffer with increased difficulties to meet financial contracts. It will be important to act swiftly in order to avoid any disruptions in the chain of payments and too much risk-averse behavior. We will fall into the 2nd Great Depression if the actions are not taken promptly and the financial world goes into the default.

It is also important to emphasize that financial regulators should refrain from relaxing critical regulatory and supervisory safeguards during this period of the pandemic. Weakening financial stability rules for large banking institutions would undermine the core resiliency of the financial system and increase risk to the real economy.

Finally, as the Covid-19 pandemic advances and other deadly viruses as bad or even worse than the Covid-19 being manufactured in the lab by weak countries, it will be optimal to aim for international cooperation on economic policy matters, including financial policy and with the coordinated responses it will lower the likelihood of "Beggar-Thy-Neighbor" policies and accusations of currency manipulation. The term "Beggar-Thy-Neighbor" is an economic policy through which one country attempts to remedy its economic problems by means tend to worsen the economic problems of other countries (Wikipedia, 2020).

With the spread of the Covid-19 many countries such as the United States are facing a potential "Black Swan Event" with extremely rare and unpredictable events that has potentially severe consequences. Therefore, it is important to act swiftly and in meaningful ways to minimize the fallout from this shock. The term "Black Swan Event" was popularized by Nassim Nicholas Taleb (2004), a finance professor, writer, and former Wall Street trader. Taleb (2004) wrote about the idea of a black swan event in a 2007 book prior to the events of the 2008 financial crisis. Taleb argued that because black swan events are impossible to predict due to their extreme rarity yet have catastrophic consequences for economy, it is important for people to plan ahead accordingly and to always assume a black swan event in any events especially in the event of an attack by a deadly virus.

The U.S. government had implemented number of massive financial measures in order to boost the economy in 2020. In mid-May 2020, the U.S. House of Representative passed the "Heroes Act", the fifth legislative effort to provide direct financial relief to small businesses, unemployed workers, healthcare professionals, first responders and more. The "Heroes Act" was a massive financial bill that was needed to address a massive challenge to the American economy and the public health system and it helped set the course towards a stronger, faster economy recover. The bill was crafted to respond to a truly unprecedented financial challenge of which the U.S. has not faced in generations. According to the Federal Reserve Administration, "Face down the challenge with bold action now, or shrink from the moment and pay the greater cost slowly over time"

It is always a good time for the U.S. Federal Reserve to spend money and deficit spending at the time of an attack with an outbreak of a pandemic disease or a deadly virus. With the current low interest rates makes it easy for the U.S. government to finance itself while limiting the potency of further monetary stimuli from the U.S. Federal Reserve. Therefore, it is incumbent upon the U.S. federal government to provide fiscal stimulus programs to ignite economic activity and that could be done in multiple times. In other words, the U.S. government needs to engage in sizeable spending and investment in key areas of the economy in order to increase economic activity and recovery; minimize disruption to the health and prosperity of the population and to limit the effects on supply chains and boost the economy and the business sectors.

The principles for economic policy action mentioned above will provide a roadmap for meaningful and decisive fiscal action that will help the economy regain its footing to certain extend during the pandemic and be prepared for any other future viruses as deadly as Covid-19 and even worse.

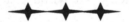

Global Impact

The worldwide disruption that was caused by the Coronavirus pandemic has resulted in numerous impacts on the global scale and environment. Countries all over the world have suffered tremendously and caused chaos and hardship and uncertainty.

Following the progression of the outbreak to new hotspot countries, people from Italy (the first country in Europe to experience a serious outbreak of the Covid-19) were also subjected to suspicion and xenophobia, as were people from hotspots in other countries. Paris has seen riots break out over police treatment of ethnic minorities during the Coronavirus lockdown (France 24, 2020). Racism and xenophobia towards

South Asians and Southeast Asians increased in the U.S., EU

countries and the Arab states of the Persian Gulf such as

Dubai, Abu Dhabi and others (Migrant Rights, 2020).

Reports from February 2020 (when most cases were

confined to China) documented racist sentiments expressed

in groups worldwide about Chinese people deserving the

virus (Bangkok Post, 2020). Citizens in countries including

Malaysia, New Zealand, Singapore, Japan, Vietnam, and South

Korea lobbied to ban Chinese people from entering their

countries (The Wall Street Journal, 2020). Chinese people and

other Asians in the United Kingdom and United States have

reported increasing levels of racist abuse and assaults. The U.S.

president Donald Trump has been criticized China multiple

times and referring to the Coronavirus as the "Chinese

Virus", which critics said it was racist and anti-Chinese

(Reuters, 2020).

In retaliation, in China discrimination and racism against non-Chinese residents has been inflamed by the pandemic with foreigners described as "foreign garbage" and targeted for "disposal" (ABC News, 2020). Some black people in China were evicted from their homes by police and told to leave China within 24 hours, due to disinformation that they and other foreigners were spreading the virus. Chinese racism and xenophobia was criticized by foreign governments and diplomatic corps and China apologized for discriminatory practices such as restaurants excluding black customers, although these and other accusations of harassment, discrimination and eviction of black people in China continued (LA Times, 2020).

Misinformation has been propagated by celebrities and politicians including heads of state in countries such as the United States, Iran, Brazil and other prominent public figures

commercial scams have claimed to offer at-home remedies and

tests for Coronavirus and supposed preventives and "miracle"

cures (The Guardian, 2020).

Several religious groups have claimed their faith will

protect them from the virus. Some even provided liquid

solutions in addition to pray to cure the Coronavirus for

a fee. Some people have claimed that the virus is a bio-

weapon accidentally or purposefully leaked from a laboratory,

a population control scheme, the result of a spy operation

(Ghaffary, 2020).

On February 10 of 2020 the Chinese government

launched a radical campaign described by paramount leader

and Chinese Communist Party general secretary as a "People's

War" to contain the viral spread (Xie, 2020). In China the

government put an order to execute "the largest quarantine

in human history" (Kang, 2020). In France referred to as

"Cordon Sanitaire" effect. It translates to draw a ring around an affected geographical area to stop the broader spread of a virus. The government of China had stopped travel in and out of Wuhan then extended to fifteen (15) Hubei cities affecting about 57 million people in 23 January 2020 and also banned all private vehicle transportation in and out of the same cities (Xiao, 2020).

In other countries, the introduction of the virus to Central and South America was largely due to international travel by the more affluent. Rapid spread resulted from an overburdened healthcare system and lack of testing and a large impoverished population many of whom live in very close proximity and are unable to socially distance or stop work. Even previous to the introduction of the Coronavirus their healthcare systems were strained and they are on the verge of being completely overwhelmed due to the Covid-19 pandemic.

In opposed to South America, Taiwan has won worldwide praise for its quick and effective Covid-19 response, which included stringent quarantines, contact tracing and widespread distribution of masks. (CNBC, 2020). Taiwan has a population of 23.7 million and is just 100 miles from China but has confirmed only 489 coronavirus cases and seven deaths (as of September 2020). Experts gave the Taiwan high point of positive 9.25 out of 10 for its handling of the pandemic. CNBC said that Taiwan's government was prepared for Covid-19 because it learned from the SARS scare of 2003. Its digital healthcare record system also enabled effective monitoring of potential high-risk patients based on travel history and Taiwanese health officials also held regular briefings to inform the public.

Opposite to Taiwan, lack of medical supplies and medical equipment has put the lives of front-line workers at risk in many countries. Furthermore, the disease is rapidly spreading from urban areas to favelas and other outlying communities and remote indigenous communities in many countries where healthcare is almost nonexistent.

It was reported that Brazil had a record 134,17 deaths in a single day and almost 18,000 fatalities in total in May 2020. With a total number of 5,122,846 cases, Brazil became the country with the third-highest number of cases (as of September 15, 2020), following Russia and the United States (Reuters, 2020).

According to BBC News, "Early detection is vital because the continent's health systems are already overwhelmed by many ongoing disease outbreaks" (2020). Social lockdowns has inflicted enormous hardship on those who depend on income earned day by day to feed themselves and their families. Because of the pandemic many countries and regions imposed quarantines and entry bans or other restrictions either for citizens and travelers to affected areas (Australian Gov., 2020). Global travel ban with decreased willingness to travel had a tremendous economy and social impact on the world travel sector such as airlines, hotels and car rentals. Concerns have been raised over the effectiveness of travel restrictions to contain the spread of Covid-19 (Nsikan, 2020).

Several countries such as the United States evacuated their citizens and diplomatic staff from affected areas in China and primarily through chartered flights of the home-based country with Chinese authorities providing clearance. Canada, Japan, India, Sri Lanka, Australia, France, Argentina, Germany and Thailand were among the first to plan the evacuation of their citizens (Tempo News, 2020). Brazil and New Zealand also evacuated their own nationals in addition to their diplomats and their families (Stuff Co., 2020).

The Netherlands, Spain, Turkey, Georgia, and the Czech Republic expressed concerns over Chinese-made masks and test kits (Fox News, 2020). It has been claimed that these materials were made in China with defects, Spain withdrew 58,000 Chinese-made Coronavirus testing kits with an accuracy rate of 30%, while the Netherlands recalled 600,000 Chinese face masks which were said to be defective (The Guardian, 2020), yet this could have been due to low quality and defected products made in China. Belgium recalled 100,000 unusable masks, which were made in China (The Brussels Times, 2020). The Philippines stopped using test kits donated by China due to their 40% accuracy (Luna, 2020). The Chinese government said product instructions might not have been followed and that some products were not purchased directly from certified companies (Global Times, 2020). Turkey provided the largest amount of humanitarian aid to the world while ranking third worldwide in supplying medical aid (Sanal Basin, 2020).

Lack of early warning, insufficient data and lack of transparency from the Chines government and their healthcare systems caused a major delay in preventing the spread of the Covid-19 pandemic globally. This is very similar to the lack precautionary warning in earlier SARS virus from China (The Guardian, 2020). The actual warning for the Coronavirus came from the WHO (World Health Organization) on January 2020 to declare the outbreak a Public Health Emergency of International Concern (PHEIC) warning that "all countries should be prepared for containment, including active surveillance, early detection, isolation and case management, contact tracing, testing and prevention of onward spread" of the virus (Kennedy, 2020).

UN (United Nation) Crisis Management Team was activated allowing coordination of the entire United Nations which the WHO stated will allow them to "focus on the health response while the other agencies could bring their expertise to bear on the wider social, economic and developmental implications of the outbreak" (WHO, 2020).

WHO (World Health Organization) officials said the Coronavirus threat assessment at the global level would be raised from "high" to "very high". This is the highest level of alert and risk assessment (CNBC, 2020). The outbreak is a major destabilizing threat to the global economy. It is forecasted that global markets and economy will remain volatile until a clearer image emerges on potential outcomes.

The effect on global economic output as a result of the pandemic is clearly demonstrated by countries like Italy, where electricity consumption has dropped as businesses shut down amid the quarantine. The huge reduction of tourist numbers and commuting workers in the city may also be leading to an improvement in the air and water quality due to a reduction of sewage discharges into the canals. Improvement in air and water resulted by the Coronavirus are the only good things about the virus.

Tourism in many countries and globally has been one of the worst affected sectors due to travel bans, closing of public places including travel attractions, and advice of governments against travel. Numerous airlines have cancelled flights due to lower demand; as a result airlines have gone bankrupt. British regional airline <u>Flybe</u> (an airline that provided more than half of UK domestic flights outside London) collapsed and bankrupt (BBC, 2020). The cruise line industry was hard hit and defined to be a good source of spreading the virus. Several train stations and ferry ports have also been closed at the global scale (Reuters, 2020). International mail between countries stopped or was delayed due to reduced transportation between them or suspension of domestic service (Cherney, 2020).

The retail sector has been impacted globally, with reductions in store hours or temporary closures. Visits to retailers in Europe and Latin America declined by 40%. North America and Middle East retailers saw a 50% to 60% drop. This also resulted in a 33% to 43% drop in foot traffic to shopping centers globally (Aislelabs, 2020).

Shopping mall operators around the world imposed additional measures, such as masks enforcement, increased sanitation, installation of thermal scanners to check the temperature of shoppers, and cancellation of events (Aislelabs, 2020).

Due to the pandemic hundreds of millions of jobs was lost globally (Al Jazeera, 2020). Nearly 48 million Americans lost their jobs and applied for government aid (BBC News, 2020). According to a UNECLA (United Nations Economic Commission for Latin America) estimate, the pandemic induced recession could leave 14 to 22 million more people in extreme poverty in Latin America than would have been in that situation without the pandemic (Fariza, 2020). The Coronavirus fears have led to panic buying of household essentials across the world, including dried and/or instant noodles, bread, rice, vegetables, and disinfectant and rubbing alcohol. India with high rate of unemployment of 23.9% of its total population of 1.3 billion is continuing with relaxing lockdown restrictions that were imposed in late March 2020. The government India of announced a $266 billion stimulus package in May 2020, but consumer demand and manufacturing are yet to recover. India's total coronavirus cases is closing in on the United States' highest tally of more than 6,687,024 million cases in compare to India total cases of 5,020,359 (16 September 2020). It is expected to surpass U.S. within weeks.

The outbreak has been blamed for several instances of supply shortages, stemming from globally increased usage of equipment to fight outbreaks, panic buying which in several places led to shelves being cleared of grocery essentials such as food, toilet paper, and bottled water and disruption to factory and logistic operations (USA Today, 2020). The technology industry, in particular, has warned of delays in shipments of electronic goods. The impact of the Coronavirus outbreak was worldwide in many respects. The pandemic has disrupted global food supplies and threatens to trigger a new food crisis (Torero, 2020). According to BBC, "We could be facing multiple famines of biblical proportions within a short few months." (2020).

OPEC (Organization of the Petroleum Exporting Countries) "scrambled" after a steep decline in oil prices due to lower demand from China (Reed, 2020). The price of West Texas Intermediate (WTI) went negative and fell to a record low (minus $37.63 a barrel) due to traders' offloading holdings so as not to take delivery and incur storage costs (BBC, 2020).

Across the world and to varying degrees, museums, libraries, performance venues and other cultural institutions had been indefinitely closed with their exhibitions, events and performances cancelled or postponed because of the pandemic. In response there were intensive efforts to provide alternative services through digital platforms (Hadden, 2020). On-line concerts, remote performances were the new norm during the pandemic.

Holy Week of Easter observances in Rome (April 12, 2020), which occur during the last week of the Christian penitential season of Lent, were cancelled (Burke, 2020). Many dioceses have recommended older Christians stay home rather than attend Mass in churches on Sundays. Services are available via radio, online live streaming and television (Fox News, 2020). All other religious bodies also cancelled services and limited public gatherings in churches, mosques, synagogues and temples (Burke, 2020). Iran's Health Ministry announced the cancellation of Friday prayers (after 41 years) in areas affected by the outbreak and shrines were later closed (Gambrell, 2020), while Saudi Arabia banned the entry of foreign pilgrims as well as its residents to holy sites in Mecca and Medina (Al Omran, 2020).

The Coronavirus pandemic has caused the most significant disruption to the worldwide sporting calendar since the Second

World War. Most major sporting events have been cancelled or postponed. Especially a big blow to the soccer fans in Europe and also to American football and basketball fans. The outbreak disrupted plans for the 2020 Summer Olympics that supposed to take place in Japan and has been rescheduled to a date beyond 2020 but not later than summer 2021 (The Guardian, 2020). For the first time since the Second World War, the Rose Parade in Pasadena, California will not be held as previously scheduled for Jan. 1, 2021 due to the pandemic.

The entertainment industry and Hollywood has also been affected; with many music groups suspending or cancelling concert tours (Associated Press, 2020). Talk shows with audiences have been move to home-based shows. Many large theaters such as Broadway shows in New York and London suspended all performances. The pandemic has affected the political systems of multiple countries, causing suspensions of legislative activities, isolations or deaths of multiple politicians, and rescheduling of elections due to fears of spreading the virus (The New York Times, 2020).

The outbreak prompted calls for the United States to adopt social health policies common in many EU countries that include universal healthcare, universal child care, paid sick leave, and higher levels of funding for public health. Political analysts anticipated that the pandemic may affect Donald Trump's chances of re-election in the 2020 presidential election (Haberman, 2020). Spreading the Coronavirus by Chinese may have been to interrupt the U.S. election and create a panic and chaos for the 2020 presidential election. There were protests in several U.S. states against government-imposed business closures and restricted personal movement and isolations. That may have contributed to riots and chaos in many states in the USA in addition to police brutality.

The Iranian government has been heavily affected by the virus, with about two dozen parliament members and fifteen current or former political figures infected (National Review, 2020). On March 2020 Iran's President Hassan Rouhani wrote a public letter to world leaders asking for help, saying they were struggling to fight the outbreak due to the lack of access to international markets from the United States sanctions against Iran (Reuters, 2020). Saudi Arabia, which launched a military intervention in Yemen in March 2020, declared a ceasefire.

Some countries have passed emergency legislation in response to the Coronavirus pandemic. Some commentators have expressed concern that it could allow governments to strengthen their grip on power (The Guardian, 2020). In the Philippines, lawmakers granted president Rodrigo Duterte temporary emergency powers during the pandemic (BBC,

2020). In Hungary, the parliament voted to allow the prime minister, Viktor Orbán, to rule by decree indefinitely, suspend parliament as well as elections, and punish those deemed to have spread false information about the virus and the government's handling of the crisis (CNN, 2020). In some countries, including Egypt, Turkey, and Thailand, opposition activists and government critics have been arrested for allegedly spreading fake news about the pandemic (The Straits Times, 2020).

In many countries, the first round of layoffs has been particularly acute in the services sector, including retail, hospitality and tourism, where women are over represented. The situation is worse in developing countries where the vast majority of women's employment is in the informal economy with few protections against dismissal or for paid sick leave and limited access to social protection (UN, April 2020).

To earn a living women as minority workers often depend on government economic support and social interactions, which are now being restricted to contain the spread of the pandemic.

As women take on greater care demands at home, their jobs will also be disproportionately affected by cuts and layoffs because of the pandemic. Such impacts risk rolling back the already fragile gains made in female labor force participation in recent years, limiting women's ability to support themselves and their families, especially for single mothers and female as head of household. Before the Covid-19 became a universal pandemic, women were doing three times as much for homecare, childcare and domestic work as men. School closures have put additional strain and demand on homemakers. According to UNESCO, 1.52 billion students and over 60 million teachers are at home as Covid-19 school closures expand. As formal and informal supply of childcare providers, homecare centers and elderly facilities decline, the demand for unpaid childcare provision is falling more heavily on women, not only because of changing the existing structure of the workforce, but also because of new social order. This will constrain women's ability to work, particularly when jobs cannot be carried out remotely. In general, women are holding 78% of all hospital jobs, 70% of pharmacy jobs and 51% of grocery store roles in the U.S. the same percentages may exist for all other countries (UN, 2020).

With children out of school and greater need of care for older persons and overwhelmed health services the price for having a homecare is much greater now than ever before. As the Covid-19 pandemic deepens economic and social stress coupled with restricted social movement and social isolation measures, gender-based violence is increasing exponentially. Many women are being forced to lockdown at home with their abusers at the same time the services to support survivors are being disrupted or made inaccessible. Women are the backbone of recovery in every community. It will be important to apply an intentional gender lens to the design of fiscal stimulus packages and social assistance programs to achieve greater equality, opportunities, and social justice and protection. According to UN "Emerging evidence on the impact of Covid-19 suggests that women's economic and productive lives will be affected disproportionately and differently from men".

Many governments started to close schools because of the pandemic. School closures impact not only students, teachers, and families but have far-reaching economic and societal consequences. School closures in response to the pandemic have shed light on various social and economic issues, including student debt, on-line learning and food insecurity as well as access to childcare, health care, housing, internet, and disability services. The impact was more severe for disadvantaged children and their families, causing interrupted learning, compromised nutrition, childcare problems, and consequent economic cost to families who could not work.

The pandemic has had many impacts on global health beyond those caused by the pandemic disease itself. It has led to a reduction in hospital visits for other illnesses. There have been 38% fewer hospital visits for heart attack symptoms in the United States and 40% fewer in Spain (Garcia, 2020). The head of cardiology at the University of Arizona said, "My worry is some of these people are dying at home because they're too scared to go to the hospital." (McFarling, 2020). There is also concern that people with strokes and appendicitis are not seeking timely treatment. Shortages of medical supplies in many countries have impacted people with various conditions and none-Covid patients.

Because of the pandemic we may have taken our attention of what we have been focusing on for years and that is "de-carbonization". Due to the pandemic we may not feel more empowered to take on daunting issues like climate change and a transition to sustainable energy sources. But in spite of any actions by human toward the climate change, the reactions of atmospheric change have been positive. The Covid-19 lockdown had led to cleaner air and fewer usage of fossil fuel combustion. There has been a lot of talk about how emissions from fossil fuel combustion have dropped radically in many countries during 2020 because of the pandemic. In the long run, cleaner air for a few months may be a tiny silver lining to Covid-19's dark clouds, but will do little in the long run to solve the problem of outdoor air pollution that kills more

than four million people every year. According to Weform.
org (2020) during the SARS outbreak in China researchers
have found that patients with SARS were more than twice as
likely to die from the disease if they came from areas of high
pollution. The same seems true for Covid-19.

In near term, the impacts of Covid-19 on the health of
the ocean have largely been positive due to the reduction in
various sectoral pressures that lead to pollution, overfishing,
habitat loss, invasive species introductions and the impacts
of climate change on the ocean. There have been significant
reductions in demand for variety of fish. This is due to lower
demand from export markets, the challenge of practicing
sanitary measures on fishing boats, difficulties accessing
supplies and labor shortage. In the U.S. two-third of
commercial fish goes to restaurants, many of which are closed
due to the pandemic and this lower demand has plummeted.

According to CNN News; "hard economic times could undermine enthusiasm for environmental protection as people prioritize health, safety, and recovery. For example, if consumers turn their backs on solar and electric vehicles, the pandemic could stem the progress we have been making toward de-carbonization".

In general the Coronavirus pandemic has resulted tremendous damage to global economy and financial system and impacted millions of people in many ways on the global scale. From environmental damage to individual wellbeing the damage is countless. Enormous damage to social structure and as a result people have suffered tremendously by the pandemic and through interruptions, chaos and hardship and uncertainty.

Workplace of the Future

The DNA of today's workplace has been changed due to the Coronavirus pandemic. The pandemic have been generating new approaches to the workplace across the globe. From lean, agile, collaborative and iterative work environment to basically remote and on-line silo working environment. Working teams across the globe have been applying different work methods to overcome the pandemic and to get the job done. Adapting to the changing world of work is a balance of getting used to or to fall behind. The workplace of the future require a whole new work arrangements, particularly in a dynamic economy characterized by high rates of job dislocation as well as job creation. It arises from workers concern both about being displaced losing a job and about

having difficulty finding another equally desirable one.

In the wake of the Covid-19 pandemic many companies

have decided to make work from home a permanent option

for their employees. Remote work offers benefits to employees

and employers alike. Some of these firms may attempt to force

those remote workers to take a pay cut of some sort. It is

an open question how those workers will react to lower pay.

Facebook was one of the first tech giants to announce that

its employees would no longer have to head into the office

on daily basis. With the number of Covid-19 cases in flux

across the U.S. and season change the work from home

workforce now appears more permanent than ever with many

companies not expecting to bring employees back until end

of 2021 and possibly beyond. As employees settle into the

reality of home office work, the conversation about security those employees protecting their data and guarding against threats both external as well as internal needs to be part of an organization's long-term planning. While many organizations excelled at getting employees the equipment and resources they needed, a long-term work from home situation for employees requires serious strategic thinking about how organizations can provide security to their staff at a time when cyber threats are increasing and cyber criminals and hackers have a bigger attack surface to target. Cyber criminals are ready to use this time in the middle of pandemic to prey on employees and businesses alike. Going beyond separating work from personal network traffic and data organizations should focus on a wide range of improvements to ensure security for the long-term including network security system audits, remote device management and user access privileges. Many organizations have used the Covid-19 pandemic to invest in an array of cloud services and giving employees access to the applications in the cloud they need to work efficiently from home.

The workplace of the tomorrow will, of course, bring new challenges during and after the pandemic. Less people than ever will work in offices and remote virtual offices will replace traditional office spaces. A growing number of people around the world will be spending less time in actual workplaces; they rather work in a virtual office or the satellite office for that matter. They will have more time on their hands to spend with their family. Their free time has been caused by massive job lost or involuntary forced to give up their jobs because of a deadly pandemic. It is a vicious cycle of madness, in one hand workers need to work to make ends meet, in other hand the killer virus is live and active ready to attack. So many forced to line up for unemployment benefits because of the job lost. Massive unemployment of a kind unknown to history has occurred in 2020. As a result the chances of developing a compassionate and caring society and a world view based on rebuild and transformation of the human spirit will be unlikely or may take a long time. In fact the pandemic has virtually transformed the nature of our society and forced us to create a new workplace of the future. This transformation affected the core fabric of businesses in a very difficult way that may take years to recover.

Organizations in their own interests and the wise companies must work with a new way of conducting business and collaboratively to make the business relation as beneficial to them as possible, but the benefits of this new work arrangement will be different from the old ones. Some of the giant technology companies like Google, Facebook, and others in Silicon Valley, California have adapted to remote workplace indefinitely for their employees. Other companies around the world have adapted social distancing in offices that will be the new norm in organizations and that is due to the Coronavirus pandemic. They need to inhere in the nature of the work itself and conducting business remotely and work in satellite offices (public WiFi access) or home-based offices. This will eliminate the need for add-ons benefits like free lunch and on-site gem or child care centers in the workplace.

When workers are working on-line and remote they must manage their time and act like unsupervised individuals in their home-based offices by maintaining a plan for career-long self-development, by taking primary responsibility for investing more quality time with their families and by renegotiating their compensation arrangements with the organization when organization goes through changes because of the pandemic and restrictions that come with it. Employees subject to new working arrangements may well react maliciously due to limited hours, lowered compensation, reduced promotion opportunities and even expectation of redundancy. These concerns at work from home can be compounded by increased levels of stress outside of the actual on-site work environment due to worries about the health of their families, livelihood and uncertainly about the future. Under these conditions, employees might become resentful or disgruntled towards the organization resulting in occurrences of information leakage and theft of intellectual property (IP).

Because more and more of the organization's efforts are likely to be undertaken by on-line connectivity and remote communications, project teams must be made up of individuals from different regions and different countries with different functional backgrounds with the capabilities of being able to switch their focus rapidly from one task to another and to work with people on-line remotely without boarders globally with very different mindsets.

Long-term employment should be for most workers, a thing of the past. The organization must recognize that they are in a difficult work environment caused by pandemic. Social distancing will be continued and to be enforced in order to effectively and gradually minimize the spread of the virus both in the social settings, family gathering and in the workplace. But all parties will have to make their long-term plans with the likelihood of such shifts in mind.

Recognizing that the pandemic has changed the fabric of business organizations, new and difficult demands have risen in every sector of business functions. Social distancing has a lot to do with this change in organizations. Individuals and organizations need to do their part in preventing the spread of the virus and providing information on critical areas and in some cases, providing training and counseling to individuals

in the workplace who are making this difficult transition from

the old rules to the new rules. Ultimately it is the responsibility

of each country's government to set the rules and enforce

them.

A surge in business organization and working from home

may lead to changes in people's long-term habits or a loss of

services in some relatively cleaner forms of transport. The

strategic imperative of timely anticipation and speedy response

to change will require the design of organizations with the

capacity to do everything safely and more carefully at the same

time faster to bring the products to market.

The faster opening the economy and businesses, the faster

financial recovery, the faster opening the economy the faster

spreading the virus, so the balance between opening the

economy and stopping the virus from spreading is a fine line and needs to be calculated so that they balance each other out. The ability to configure the organization in a new way that ensures a constant and acute awareness of impending changes in the workplace will become an essential capability that will separate the leaders from the laggards. Beyond that, organizations and leaders will have to find creative ways to achieve unprecedented speed in getting the right workers without the boarders and setup all their organizational operating tools and standardize business processes in era of the pandemic as they want to significantly reduce their time to market and time to volume in the form of new supply chain format.

Leaders should accelerate decision-making up and down the line and they need to substantially cut the time it takes to design and implement strategic and organizational changes in order to cope with the challenges caused by the Covid-19 pandemic and future deadly viruses. Enlightened leaders already understand that speed does not mean operating the same way as in the past before the pandemic, but only safer and faster combined to bring the products to consumers; they know that radical improvements in speed for better supply chain involve doing things much safer and a lot different in many ways of business management.

Leaders of tomorrow will soon realize to implement the use of PPE (Personal Protective Equipment) supplies in the work environment. Equipment such as masks, hand satirizers, protective gloves, face shields, clothing's (in some places) and other medical equipment that will be essential in the workplace to fight not only the Covid-19 pandemic and future viruses as deadly as the Coronavirus. Providing worker's protective gears should be an essential part of any organizations in longer term. Future organizations should have a safety department with safety committee to inforce safety regulations in respect to the pandemic and future deadly viruses alike.

The government must play a far different role in eliminating the pandemic. One in every four people has died because of this pandemic in 2020. Governments that were less tied to the interests of the people, their health had suffered with the greater loss of lives one example is the USA. In average 900 people were dying every day in the United States during the 2nd quarter of 2020 and since the pandemic has entered into the country. Those governments that were more aligned with the interests of the people and their social health has definitely suffered less, like Thailand.

There are millions of foreign workers in the U.S. on work visas. These workers are either from India for IT work or from Mexico for agricultural and farming jobs. The U.S.

government has changed immigration policies for foreign workers to let the U.S. citizens to have a better chance and high priority in finding jobs that are being taken by Asian-Indian workers in high paying IT jobs. Giving the U.S. citizens and U.S. workers first priority and the opportunity in getting high paying IT jobs is a moral obligation of every American leader, rather than organizations saving few buck in hiring cheap foreign labors who are living in their suitcases and having high paying IT jobs. Thanks to the Whitehouse for the new immigration package that included several other long-sought changes to the H-1B visa programs, including narrowing the definition of qualifying specialty occupations and placing more requirements on companies hiring these foreign workers as contractors mostly Asian-Indians.

The administration has shorten the length of H-1B visas for foreign workers who had paid at the lowest pay tier and required companies to pay increases for them upon INS renewal. Another INS proposal policy has been the elimination of work permits for asylum seekers, a move that the U.S. government had already formally proposed along with refugees and other immigrants.

Less foreign workers employment will, off course, increase the chances for the American workers to take high paying IT jobs and bring the unemployment down in the U.S.A and also rebuild new immigration regulations in order to better control the flukes of workers coming to the U.S. from countries like India, Mexico Philippine and Central America.

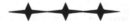

Inventing Tomorrow

Social structures throughout much of past century were generally viewed as a way to institutionalize and manage stability. But today in the Covid-19 pandemic era, the challenge is to design social structures that are flexible and adaptive to change. New social structures should be able to perform effectively in the face of uncertainty not just day-to-day but in the broader context of profound continuous change. New strategic imperatives create a corresponding set of challenges for the society and organizations of the future. As far as the organization change, business leaders should be forced to become proficient in a few core competencies such as safety in the workplace, elimination of discrimination, new policies and procedures to better manage deadly viruses and safer workplace configurations. Organizations should be providing new operating tools and platforms for workers for better and faster supply chain.

Tomorrow may look different than today but the challenge is who will make tomorrow better than it has been. That may require a change not only cross the society and economy but the business environment and the government itself. Other concern is the impact of a newer and deadlier virus near future. Some believe the Covid-19 pandemic has been deadly and has been worse than SARS, but future deadlier viruses supposed to be more difficult to control and manage and will be more deadlier. Business environment and challenges ahead will shape our fundamental assumptions of doing business a lot different and redesigning organizational culture to cope with these kinds of disasters. Changing physical part of business environment is easy; changing the culture of the business is hard and time consuming. The same applies to the culture of a society.

One way to avoid the virus is to stay at home and to work remote in the comfort of the home. Working in offices may no longer be needed for many office workers, especially for IT sector. Work from home will be a new norm. Employment life cycles for the workers will be shorten drastically with the flexibility of fast turn overs and utilization of satellite office retaining global knowledge workers in a borderless and virtual working environment.

Many countries implemented strategies for preventing spread of the pandemic. Encouraging individuals to maintain social distancing, wearing face masks, maintain good personal hygiene, washing hands multiple times during the day, avoiding handshakes, avoid touching eyes, nose or mouth with unwashed hands, and coughing or sneezing into a tissue to avoid the spread of the virus. Those who may already have the infection have been advised to wear a surgical mask in public (CDC, 2020) Physical distancing measures in the workplace are also recommended to prevent transmission of the virus.

Many governments have restricted or advised against all non-essential travel to and from countries and areas affected by the outbreak. The virus has already spread within cities in large parts of the world, with many not knowing where or how they were infected (CDC, 2020). Mis-conceptions were circulating about how to prevent infection. Although there is no Covid-19 vaccine at present time, many medical organizations around the world are working hard to develop a vaccine (The Guardian, 2020). Even if the vaccine is developed the Coronavirus may stay with us for a longtime. Other deadly viruses may soon be arriving and impacting the countries the same way as Covid-19 has been. A new biological

warfare is more effective than the nuclear war.

The timely of the spread of the Coronavirus was most

definitely calculated and precisely implemented by Chinese

either deliberately or by accident. Either way the origin of

the spread of both viruses like SARS in 2003 and Covid-19

in 2019-2020 are known to be in China. The big question is

"What other deadly viruses will be coming next?" We know

the origin but we don't know when a new deadly virus will

arrive?

Prompt identification and isolation of potentially infected

individuals is a critical step in protecting public, visitors and

others in a society and in a workplace. The U.S. Centers for

Disease Control and Prevention (CDC) recommends that

employees who have symptoms of acute respiratory illness

such as the Covid-19 pandemic should stay home until they

are free of fever, signs of a fever and any other symptoms for at least 24 hours without the use of fever-reducing or other symptom-altering medicines. The sick leave policies in the workplace should be flexible and permit workers to stay home to care of themselves and/or their sick family members. These policies that are either old or recently revised must be carefully revisited and that the workers of organizations must be aware of these revised policies and that can be done through the training.

There are also psychosocial hazards for individuals that are increasing from anxiety or stress from worries about contracting the virus, or the illness or death of a relative or friend, changes in work patterns and financial or interpersonal difficulties. In some countries men commit suicide due to the lack of income and losing jobs and those who cannot pay bills and are in financial trouble. Outrage, anger, stress and anxiety are psychological issues caused by the Covid-19 pandemic for many people. These psychological problems will cause alcoholism, violence, drug abuse and other addictions.

Preventing measures such as social distancing and personal space will minimize the spread of the virus. The elimination of the direct contact with the family members and friends and co-workers might be a good way to stop the spread of the virus but indirect contract with family members and the love ones is essential to maintain the relationship. These might include family members checking on each other and asking how they were, facilitating family member interactions and assisting them in daily activities such as grocery shopping and preparing meals at distance.

As far as the workplace, work environments may contribute substantiality to spread of the virus and potentially expose workers to the virus as they often work close to one another or on processing lines during prolonged work shifts in manufacturing sectors. For better controls, CDC (Centers of Disease Control and Prevention) and OSHA (Occupational Safety and Health Administration) recommend configuring communal work environments so that workers are spaced out at least six feet apart along processing lines in manufacturing environment, using physical barriers such as strip curtains or Plexiglas and Clear Acrylic Sheet to separate workers from each other and ensuring adequate ventilation that minimizes air from fans blowing from one worker directly at another worker. These extra precautionary measures will cost organizations extra money that they don't have and not been budgeted. The impact of the pandemic to the organization cross a globe will be costly and will continue to drag for years and the burden of paying for it goes to consumers.

For non-manufacturing workplaces and office administrative, CDC and OSHA recommend staggering workers' arrival, break, and departure times and for cohering workers such as health care workers they should be always assigned to the same shifts with the same coworkers, encouraging single-file movement through the facility, avoiding carpooling to and from work and considering a program of screening workers before entry into the workplace and setting criteria for return to work of recovered workers and for exclusion of sick workers. These measures in preventing the spread of the Covid-19 pandemic may be affective, but learning from the exposure will help organizations to maintain the same routines in case of the next deadly virus that may appear sooner than anticipated.

According to CDC (2020) Strategies in the control of an outbreak are "Containment", "Suppression" and "Mitigation".

Containment is undertaken in the early stages of the outbreak and aims to trace and isolate those infected as well as introduce other measures of infection control and vaccinations to stop the virus from spreading to the rest of the population. Suppression requires more extreme measures so as to reverse the Covid-19 pandemic by number of restrict measures. When it is no longer possible to contain the spread of the pandemic, efforts then should be moved to the mitigation stage. Mitigation measures are taken to slow the spread and mitigate its effects on the healthcare system and society. A combination of both containment and mitigation measures may be undertaken at the same time. (NPIs, 2020).

As far as other safety measures, community measures are as important and are aimed to prevent the spread of the virus in public places such as shutting down shops, restaurants and closing schools and cancelling mass gathering sport events; community engagement to encourage acceptance and participation in such interventions as well as environmental measures like surface cleaning, public seating cleaning and disaffect germs, public transportation cleaning and other public areas (CMGPPI, 2017).

Workplaces need to be safer and healthier than ever before, but both the intractable health and safety hazards of yesterday and the unknowable hazards of tomorrow will require continued vigilance and cooperation among individual workers, employers, society, healthcare providers and the government. Preventing the spread of the virus and resolving old office problems (crowding offices, tight quarters, crowded meeting rooms) and recognizing new ones early on will also require new efforts in workplace health regulations and set new policies for preventing the spread of the Covid-19 pandemic and to develop an atmosphere of secure and safe for all workers regardless of the industry. New technologies can provide solutions to resolve many workplace safety issues such as working remotely and on-line work and work from home-based offices. Some solutions, however, are simple to provide like changing the policies and the way workers work can help to reduce the spread of the virus in the workplace and minimize illnesses and health issues. Training workers can create awareness on how to prevent the spread of the virus in the workplace.

In spite of the fact that workplaces of today are fairer than ever before, much remains to be done. While woman and some minority groups have made advances, in educational attainment, employment, sports and earnings, there are still workplaces where they are not welcoming African-American of less educated. "Tomorrow's work will place even more of a premium on workers with education and skills." (Herman,

1999, p.101). Employers cannot afford to discriminate against any levels of employees in organizations based on race or color, disability, national origin, gender, religion, sex or age. Workers deserve a safer workplace free of discrimination and racism with continued attention and support of employers and cooperation's among policymakers and the support of the government.

Historically however, African American workers have always faced unemployment rates that were about twice as high as those of white workers. The 2:1 ratio has held basically steady since 1972 when the Labor Department first started collecting data on the African American unemployment rate. The post-Coronavirus economy might widen the unemployment gap between white and Black workers even more. Black women might have an even tougher struggle going back to work because of the increased childcare burdens placed on parents. And, as state and local governments start laying off more workers to deal with budget shortfalls, those job cuts are more likely to fall on African Americans. Meanwhile, the pandemic has widened educational disparities for Black and white children. Long term that could mean worsening opportunities for those disadvantaged children when they enter the job market years from now.

As the Covid-19 pandemic has changed the social behavior of the globe and created a new norm, many organizations prefer to see a strong need for a new innovation and creation of a new workplace settings and modernization. The future workplace should have global workers without borders with considerable knowledge to achieve progress. Remote and off-site home-based offices are the workplace of the future where workers will be safe in their own homes with their family to take care of 24/7 at the same time to perform their job duties on-line. Of course some organizations may call

some of its staff back to work, with focus on those employees

who simply were not capable of doing their jobs from home,

either due to the requirements of their work or simply

because their home environments have not been conductive

to getting things done. Those people who return to work

should continue to focus on social distancing and limiting

interpersonal contact as much as possible, even to the point

of restricting the number of people who should be allowed

to travel in a single elevator at the same time. In spite of all

these restrictions and regulations many workers would not be

returning to work for at least several years (cycle of 7 years).

Employees should be strongly encouraged by companies to

take on-site or at home virus tests that companies should be

providing to staff members. High tech companies like Google,

Facebook and Twitter can afford to bide their time as it is

much easier for software engineers to work from home and

from anywhere.

There should not be any needs for on-site office workers

jamming together in organizations, or global business settings

and crowding offices. Advisors, consultants, employees and

executives of the future should be able to work together via

satellite offices and remotely on-line to conduct meetings via

high tech applications. Furthermore, remote working should

be the way of the future for many of workers and we all

should get used to it.

Another area that left wide open for the U.S. workers

is the replacement of foreign workers in the United States.

Labor market experts believe that foreign workers on work

visa no longer needed to be on site in America. 95% of them

are high tech office workers and they don't need to be on-site

to work in the United States. They can work from anywhere

24/7 globally. Some organizations in the U.S. and elsewhere are practicing this working model at present time without the actual need for on-site office setup, kind of office-less workers. Organizations want to become more efficient in producing results and workers want to protect themselves against many negative elements such as layoffs, economy downfall, and deadly viruses like the Covid-19.

Future remote workers with advanced software applications will not have any problems performing their jobs with unlimited time to spend at home office both during the business hours and also off hours to accomplish what they are supposed to accomplish for the business. Business communication will not be limited to 8 to 5 working hours but 24/7. These changes in the workplace are the new way of the future for many global high tech companies and organizations.

Certainly changing the organizational culture from what it has been to what need to be is hard to achieve. Workers and organizations should learn how to cope with health issues and unknown deadly viruses of the future. There is a growing policy division regarding the new workplace of the future. Some perceive this new remote workforce will not work for manufacturing and auto makers and many other similar industries. The debate whether to go remote or on-site for companies across the globe yet need to be discussed by business leaders.

The employers should delegate tasks and responsibilities to remote off-site workers with no benefits, little or no mutual loyalty and all risk borne by the employers would be minimized while remote workers benefit from lower costs of work commute and travel expenses borne by the employees. The high cost of obtaining work visa for foreign workers has been borne by the U.S. employers for many years. INS has been over loaded with visa petitions and extensions and applications approval for permanent residency (Green Card) for these foreign workers.

In recent months in 2020 the U.S. Courts and Congress have passed new policies in reforming immigration laws for foreign workers in the United States. One example of immigration reform is barring relatives of the U.S. permanent residents, American citizens' parents and diversity visa winners from entering the U.S., but exempting foreign investors, the U.S. citizens' spouses and their minor children and healthcare workers.

According to INS (2020) due to the Covid-19 pandemic and staff reduction in immigration and Naturalization Service employers will no longer need to submit client letters or purchase orders for H-1B workers and the USCIS (United

States Citizenship and Immigration Services) will not require

to prove specific work assignments for duration of the H-1B

petition. This may be a win-win situation both for the workers

and also for the employers but there is a negative side to

this. Overwhelming work load for Fed employees to take

care of foreign workers visa will lead to INS workers being

furloughed and INS employees forced to take the leave of

absence or temporary release from their job because of the

pandemic, the same applies to IRS (Internal Revenue Service)

and all other U.S. Federal departments.

Another INS policies change were for all new H-1B

visa holders specialty occupation worker applications be

banned unless the worker pays at the highest wage level-4

(Level-4: salary range $150,000 to $250,000 or more a

year). New immigration policies mandated to suspend all

new L1 visa (business owners, employees who had worked

for a U.S. company outside the U.S. for one year to 3 years)
intracompany transferees such as international executives,
managers, workers with advanced or specialized knowledge.
The new policies of INS also suspend all new H-2B visas
for temporary non-agricultural workers unless the work is
essential to the maintenance of the USA food supply chain.
These INS new policies further needed to reform the U.S.
immigration policies.

In the U.S. 2020 presidential election Joe Biden's party
has made history by unveiling the nation's first Black vice
presidential nominee Kamala Harris in August 2020. She
is the child of immigrants; her mother immigrated to the
United States from India and her father from Jamaica. As a
Black woman she understands how systemic racism keeps
many African-Americans from succeeding and as a woman
she understands how sexism is still rampant in our nation.

Mrs. Harris as a VP should fight for economic and judicial

equality for Black and Brown people, affordable healthcare for

all and full equality for women. In spite of the fact that Mrs.

Harris is half Asian-Indian she may reverse President Trump's

immigration laws and executive orders to undo the ban of

H-1B visa workers and flood the U.S. with foreign workers if

Biden and Harris get elected to the Whitehouse. That would

be a double disaster for the U.S. to first take away American

jobs, and second to undo Trump's good works.

Another reform should be for the USA justice department

and the public policing procedures and policies. According to

recent on-line media report (2020) it is estimated that many

African-Americans are killed every day in the USA by police

brutality. According to mappingpoliceviolence.org number of

African-American that were killed in 2013 were 1,106, 1,050

killed in 2014, 1,103 killed in 2015, 1,071 killed in 2016, 1,095 killed in 2017, 1,243 killed in 2018, 1,109 killed in 2019 and

576 killed in 2020 and still counting. It is interesting to know

that 97% of the killing occurred while a police officer was

acting in a law enforcement capacity.

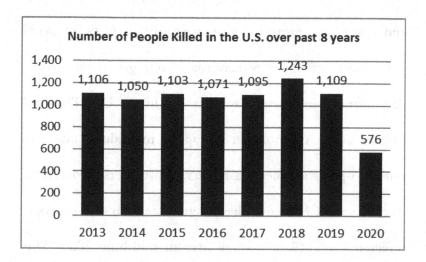

The above data has been sourced from the three largest

and most comprehensive and impartial crowd sourced

databases on police killings in the U.S.A. As a result riots

and demonstrations against these kinds of brutality and

discrimination happened from Chicago to Los Angeles and 48

other states and also all over the world from London to Hong Kong and other places.

Recent killing of George Floyd in Minneapolis sparked fury over racism and police brutality. In spite of all warnings and preventive measures that were put in place to avoid the spread of the Coronavirus, large group of people demonstrated in masses day after day in the U.S. That will further affect much larger group of individuals and will cause hospitals and healthcare service providers to overflow. According to CNN news there were more than 43,000 people infected Covid-19 in a single day in mid-June 2020. This infections surge was as a result of group demonstrations and has caused stress on healthcare providers and workers and hospitals staff dealing with large number of the Covid-19 victims. BBC News reported that Dr. Anthony Fauci mentioned the U.S. has a "Serious Problem and the only way we are going to end it is by ending it together" (June, 2020).

He further mentioned "The official number of the U.S.A.

Covid-19 infections is expected to pass 2.5 million by end of

June 2020", and it did surpass this number to 6,828,300+ by

mid-September 2020.

In addition to the public demonstrations and nationwide

protests over the recent deaths of black men and women at

the hands of police and racial injustice in America, there have

been examination of confederate symbols and monuments

in the U.S. Protesters in some states have defaced or tried

to tear down statues, denouncing them as racist symbols of

America's legacy of slavery. According to New York governor

Andrew Cuomo "You played politics with this virus and you

lost". Governor Cuomo of New York has done a great work in

bringing the number of Covid-19 cases down and that resulted

in less death in New York State (June 2020). He is considered a great communicator giving daily live report on Covid-19. Other states not so lucky and they rushed to reopen their economy and that brought the number of cases up in addition to death projections that have gone up as a result.

To address social health issues and to better control of viruses like Covid-19, policy makers need to rethink the current prevention policies and setup specific new laws to resolve mass social issues such as racism, social unrest, uprising, unemployment, and economy reform in addition to better control of future deadly viruses. These kind of deadly viruses are a new weapon of the future warfare. It is not a cold war for sure but a deadly war in fact.

Regardless of the reasons, the United States of America cannot afford to let any class of society fall behind their desire to live, work and pursue of happiness. There are classes of society that may need skill development and the training of various kinds in order to join the workforce. If these classes are motivated enough to develop their skills and join the workforce, then there should not be any needs for the foreign workers to come to the USA and take American jobs.

According to U.S. Census Bureau in 2020, it is estimated that 4.5 million Asian-Indian (18% increase than 2017 and 50% increase than 2018) workers are in the U.S. for variety of jobs, especially in the high tech industries. The U.S. has enough human resources to accommodate for the need of organizations in the U.S. rather than brining foreign workers from countries like India. It is a moral obligation of every American leader to shift their thought process in hiring American workers rather than foreign workers.

In June 2020 the Trump administration has been weighing a proposal to suspend a slate of employment-based immigration visa. That included the coveted H-1B high-skilled visa workers. According to administration officials these new measures are based on high unemployment and economic fallout of the pandemic, among several other measures. Officials further mentioned that the proposed suspension could extend into the government's new fiscal year beginning Oct 1, 2020, when many new visas are typically issued to foreign workers. That could bar any new H-1B visa holder outside the country from coming to work until the suspension is lifted. Barring H-1B visa workers could eliminate approximately 100,000 immigrants and foreign workers from the workforce over time. In addition, the administration is mulling a proposal to change the H-1B application fee to $20,000 from current fee of $460 (June, 2020) though some companies pay hundreds or thousands of dollars more in additional fees. These fees will supplement the INS budget shortfall due to the Covid-19 pandemic and overall economy downfall. INS officials said increasing H-1B visa costs could help USCIS, plug a hole in its budget. The agency which is funded through fees it collects on immigration applications was asking congress for $1.2 billion bailout.

The U.S. visa suspension proposal was one of a series of legal immigration limits that President Trump was considering as part of an executive action he had planned to implement in 2020. The administration had argued that the pandemic required limits on immigration to prevent sick people from entering the U.S. and to ensure that Americans get jobs first as the economy rebounds rather than jobs go to the foreign workers.

In addition to the suspension of H-1B visa, the suspension could apply to the H-2B visa holders for short-term seasonal workers and the suspension for the J-1 visa for short-term workers including camp counselors and the L-1 visa holders for internal company transfer. The administration planned to exempt some industries from the restrictions, such as healthcare workers that are directly involved in treading the Coronavirus patient and other critical industries to the food supply chain. The administration was also considering a broader carves-out allowing employers to hire immigrants if they could prove they could not hire Americans for a given job. Some opposition believed barring immigrants who have unique skill sets or take jobs most Americans would not perform would hamper economic growth rather than bolster it. Many Americans believe they would rather have high paying jobs especially in IT sector than giving these jobs to foreign workers like Asian-Indians. According to Republican House of Senate (2020) "American businesses that rely on help from these visa programs should not be forced to close without serious consideration. Guest workers are needed to boost American business, not to take American jobs". According to some members of special groups favoring immigration restrictions that "while the proposals echo policies they have long urged Mr. Trump to adopt, they worried he would side with businesses who oppose them" (Federation for American Immigration Reform, 2020). It is clear that some politicians are more worried about big business interests than unemployed American workers and this is the reason for having 4.5 million Asian-Indian workers in the U.S.A.

The U.S. federal government has the training programs to education American workers to take over the IT sector that is currently run by Asian-Indians. Among many training options that the U.S. government can provide to all Americans is the support of career development and the training either indirectly through diverse organizations with the capabilities to conduct such training or directly by the federal agencies. As in the support of the government at present time for the training is given by the Department of Labor (DoL) and by the Small

Business Administration (SBA) and other federal agencies.

The only president that has tried and succeeded to change

the Immigration and the INS policies in suspending foreign

workers coming to the U.S. is President Trump. In April 2020,

Trump signed an executive order that was needed to protect

American jobs. According to CNN Politics, against the

backdrop of the Coronavirus pandemic, the administration

has pressed forward with a series of immigration measures

that, prior to the Coronavirus, had struggled to break through.

Among those changes has been the closure of the southern

border to south of the boarder migrants (Central American

Countries & Mexican) including those who were seeking

asylum, unless certain conditions are met. This will fast

forward in reducing the flow of South American immigrants

coming into the United States. As unemployment remain

high some say the immigrant are important for economic recovery and the administration should allow immigrates to temporarily work in the U.S. were critical to the economy.

These complex immigration issues could not easily be resolved. While the Codiv-19 pandemic continues to spread throughout the countries, lack of jobs and the insecurity of the workers are big concerns of workers for the U.S. nationals. According to CNN, the President Trump administration has prepared roll out sets of restrictions on legal immigration, citing the impact of the Coronavirus pandemic on society and organizations causing high unemployment, in spite of the fact that he is also arguing for the reopening of the U.S. economy (2020). Despite a push from President Trump to move past the pandemic, the administration has been continuing to usher forward immigration measures, citing the outbreak and its toll on the economy.

Because of the pandemic many jobs have been eliminated and caused a panic among workers on job insecurity that included both lack of jobs, job change and workers' perceptions about future job security. Job stability can be measured in terms of how long jobs last in a new workplace with the pandemic still lingering among groups of people. Job security, however, is more subjective: workers may voluntarily change jobs more often when economic times are good or change jobs less often when they are more concerned about job security and see fewer opportunities. Involuntary job loss clearly provides one measure of job insecurity.

How much value do workers place on job security in spite of the Pandemic? While loss of jobs are generally an unpleasant experience, a highly skilled and highly mobile workforce may place a lower value on job stability and may even value voluntary job change and job variety. Concern about job security probably diminishes for many workers during the pandemic periods of high unemployment when the risk of long periods of employment is less.

Many people believe job insecurity has increased in recent years especially with the Covid-19 pandemic. Despite high unemployment rates that would seem to indicate increasing on job insecurity. The 2020 has been marked by concern about displaced workers, those who permanently lost their jobs because their job site or company closed, bankrupt or moved because of the pandemic.

In 1991 and 1992, 5.4 million workers were displaced; about half of them (2.8 million) were long-tenured workers, workers who had held their jobs for three or more years (Gardner, 1995). Labor market recovery from "the 1990–1991 recessions (George H. W. Bush presidency 1989-1993) were slow compared to recent recoveries recessions. But when economic activity accelerated in 1993 and 1994 (Bill Clinton Presidency 1993-2001), both the level and the risk of job displacement began to fall. Historically between 1993 and 1994, a period of strong labor market conditions, 2.4 million long-tenured workers were displaced from their jobs, 0.4 million fewer were displaced between 1991 and 1992 (Hipple, 1997). The displacement rate, which reflects the likelihood of job loss, fell from 3.9% in the 1991–1992 (Bush era) periods to 20% in 2020 the pandemic era. Bureau of Labor Statistics (BLS) data show that "during the 1995–1996 periods (Clinton era), the number of workers displaced fell further to 2.2 million and the displacement rate to 2.9%." (Hipple, 1999).

There is every reason to believe that once the Covid-19 pandemic is gone the jobs will return quickly. Sudden explosion of jobs opening will create huge demand for skilled workers who are capable to work off-site, on-line and remotely. The need for skilled workers will be reinforced by continuing changes in how companies and organizations operate and to increase workers autonomy. Employers of the future will place increasing value on workers who not only can operate remotely with the technology tools of tomorrow, but who also can find ways to increase their productivity remotely and increase their earnings.

As the workplaces of the future respond to deadly viruses and technological change in addition to cultural change and global competition, as well as the needs of workers who can produce without supervision and work in silo. The use of remote workforce will likely rise globally. Additionally, these workforce trends may result in declining job stability. Workers must be ready to manage the changes and dislocations they may face by keeping their skills up to date.

Road Ahead

In the Covid-19 pandemic era U.S. businesses are living in fear, they are shutting down their businesses or customers would not return. Managers are struggling to keep up with changing safety guidelines. School districts are grappling with whether to reopen schools in fall or winter of 2020. Parents are straining to juggle full-time jobs with kids at home. And supply chains are showing worrying signs of shortages of products. For many, there is a growing sense of "lost year."

As so much hangs in the balance, the bulk of the federal government aid for small businesses and unemployed has expired August 1st 2020. Congress and President Trump have been unable to come to a deal on more relief, adding to the uncertainty. The recovery is stalling on many fronts, and economists warn there's heightened risk of backsliding.

"Households and businesses are really fragile. This is not a recovery that we should be confident in," said Wendy Edelberg, director of the Hamilton Project at the Brookings Institution and former head of the commission that investigated what went wrong in the 2008 financial crisis. "Government policy is not making it better right now. Policy is exacerbating uncertainty." When uncertainty is high, it usually triggers more layoffs, less investment and more business closures. Business investment fell to the lowest level in 68 years in spring of 2020 and consumer spending has stalled in mid-2020.

The COVID-19 pandemic has disrupted life in America like few other events in living memory, and it has placed families under tremendous stress. The coronavirus and botched government response have thrown the economy into the deepest crisis since the Great Depression and the recovery has been highly unlikely. Real estate is a telling example. 40 million U.S. home owners are subject to default and eviction by fall of 2020. Home foreclosures will flood the real estate market in late 2020 with no buyers. According to MSN News (2020) in conversations with 14 small business owners and laid off workers across the country, nearly all were frustrated by the lack of clear guidelines from state and national leaders, and many were suffering personally as Congress let aid lapse at such a critical time.

The White House often points to stock market gains, which have recovered nearly all their pandemic losses as tech stocks like Apple have soared and investors believe large companies will be the most likely to survive the downturn and profit as their small competition is crushed. The federal and state governments are not doing more to help the restaurants and small shops that have clearly been hit the hardest. While employment remains down in most sectors, it is still off 25% in hospitality, which includes hotels and restaurants.

On August 3, 2020 president Trump signed an executive order to prevent federal agencies from unfairly replacing U.S. workers with lower cost and cheaper foreign labor especially in IT sector. Trump also said that he was formally removing the Tennessee Valley Authority (TVA) chairperson of the board and another member of the board and threatened to remove other board members if they keep hiring foreign labor according to MSN News. (2020). The White House and advocate groups criticized the TVA for furloughing its own workers and replacing them with contractors using foreign workers with H-1B visas. TVA outsourced 20% of its technology jobs to companies based in foreign countries.

TVA's action could cause more than 200 highly skilled American tech workers in Tennessee to lose their jobs to foreign workers hired on temporary work visa according to the White House.

In spite all the wrong things that President Trump did during his 1st administration, he has done great work in many fronts; he stopped China from unfear trading with the U.S., he pulled out to WHO that China was the head of the organization, he changed the INS for foreign workers, he pulled out of NATO, he reversed most of Obama's executive orders that benefited many minorities and had little to contribute to the U.A. society as a whole. He renegotiated the North American Trade Agreement (NAFTA) between Canada, U.S. and Mexico for better trade. The new trade agreement between the United States, Mexico, and Canada replaced the 25-year-old North American Trade Agreement

(NAFTA). He has done so much for the goodness of the United States of America, than any other president in recent years.

As we continue to learn more about biological warfare and the impact of Covid-19 pandemic on individual, society, economy and the workplace, the improper preventive measures of tomorrow killer viruses would be deadly. Only by building strong, self-sustaining local communities people will be able to withstand the forces of biological warfare and displacement and global market diminishment that are threatening the livelihoods and survival much of the human society. The government of tomorrow will have to play a far different role in the healthcare management area and create an early warning system to better control the pandemic. Government should forge a new partnership with all sectors of the society in rebuilding the social economy that could help restore civic order once a new pandemic realized.

Feeding the poor, providing healthcare services, educating the nation's youth, building affordable housing and preserving the environment tops the list of urgent priorities in years ahead. All of these critical areas have been either ignored or inadequately paid attended to by the forces of the pandemic and most likely future viruses that will continue to interrupt social order of the future.

The U.S. should not lose her position in the world as a global leader to a country like China. According to Kevin Rudd, president of the Asia Society Policy Institute and the former Australian prime minister "The global leadership vacuum during the coronavirus crisis is an "open door" for China to walk through, the U.S. has presented an opportunity for Beijing to seize global leadership during the pandemic".

From China's perspective, looking at the debacle of the U.S. domestic management of Covid-19 and the failure of the U.S. to provide global leadership and response to what is a global public health and economic crisis and then it's very difficult sitting in Beijing not to identify a leadership vacuum and to walk right into it. That comes as the U.S. is criticizing and walking away from allies and multilateral institutions like the World Trade Organization (WTO) and the World Health Organization (WHO).

The U.S. has paid to the American families through multiple simulation programs and provided financial support of billions of dollars to organizations and individuals to prepare men and women of every color in every community to return to work. These simulation programs require significant government funding. "While there would be a loss of taxable revenue at the front side, it would likely be more than compensated for by a diminished need for expensive government programs to cover needs and services best handled by volunteer efforts." (Rifkin, 1995, pp. 256-257). Some of the money could come from savings brought about by gradually replacing many of the current welfare programs set by Obama and previous administrations with direct payments to healthcare workers and the families who are in need of money to make ends meet. With community organizations and nonprofit groups taking greater responsibility for addressing needs traditionally handled by government, more tax money would be freed up to provide incomes and training for the millions young and working people and for those who would be working in their neighborhood to help others.

As far as workplace safety, workers should be better protected against viruses in the workplace. Employers can shift their budge and resources on increasing their focus on employees and providing greater opportunities for those of color and education and training, rather than paying workers' compensation for preventable injuries caused by unsafe work place.

Massive unemployment of a kind in 2020 unknown in history after the Great Depression occurred as a result of a killer virus Covid-19. The chances of developing a compassionate and caring society are slim and will take years to transform and rebuild the human spirit. We have seen the massive disastrous results of the pandemic to society. We have seen more of the negative effects of the pandemic rather than the positive side of it. The negative effects are deaths, down economy, social breakdown, jobs and business lost and many others. The positive effects of the pandemic are good air quality and less heavy traffic stress and decreased emissions of pollutants and reduction in greenhouse gases.

Another semi-positive side of the pandemic was that in the middle of the Covid-19 pandemic turmoil new generations of people transcend with the narrow limits of nationalism and begin to think and act as common members of the community bonding people regardless of the race. Neighborhood community organizations in the U.S. are very effective in doing effective work rather than the depending on government. Their solidarity and togetherness makes the U.S. unique in many ways.

If the talent, energy and resourcefulness of hundreds of millions of men and women are not redirected to constructive and positive ways during the pandemic and thereafter, civilization as we have it will probably continue to disintegrate into a state of increasing destitution, chaos and lawlessness

from which there may be no easy return or may take
generations to undo. For this reason, finding an alternative
to formulate a new social order without the discrimination,
racism and lawlessness ultimately finding a way to keep
individuals, groups, associations, communities happy is
the critical task ahead for every government and officials.
Preparing for a post-pandemic era will require far greater
attention to the building up better social economy combining
minorities of every color and every race and the renewal of
community life.

The fabric of social community is centered on human
relationships, on feelings of intimacy, on companionship,
fraternal bonds and stewardship, qualities can easily reducible
to or replaceable by fear and separation by a pandemic. This is
one realm that viruses can fully penetrate and spread quickly
to the masses, it will be by necessity the refuge where the

displaced societies of workers go to find renewed meaning and purpose in life after the commodity value of their labor in the formal marketplace has become marginal or worthless.

The path to a successful change journey is associated with systematic change processes combined with change in individual, society, government and private sectors that are not undermining the transformation efforts. Some of the recommended stages in making society change and building on the new paradigm will include number of actions from both the government and the communities. Government will allocate financial resources and communities will provide human resources. These two resources combined with new change regulations, policies and procedures will derive the change in a gradual upward to completion.

According to Spencer (1874) Society is an aggregate of individuals and change in society could take place only once the individual members of that society had changed. In other words, the change will happen by individuals and is a top-down process; the change will affect society as a whole. The society of the future will need to adapt to a new behavior to fight all obstacles and resistance and work with individuals in all levels in making the social change and to succeed and become one unit. Through individual and group training the change could gradually be implemented. Social media has a big rule in doing so. In spite of the pandemic all sectors of society starting with individuals, groups, industries and government will need to do the processes of change simultaneously in order to accommodate the need of people.

Recognizing that the pandemic has changed the fabric of society, new and difficult demands have emerged and risen in every sector of a society. Individuals, organizations and government need to do their part in preventing the spared of the today's killer virus and the deadlier viruses of tomorrow. Providing information on critical areas and in some cases providing training and counseling to people who are making this difficult transition from the old rules to the new rules. Ultimately it is the responsibility of each country's government to set the rules and enforcing them.

To make a change one needs to be motivated to make efforts to change as individual. Individual efforts in a community will create a sense of need to make a change. Community efforts to make the change will cause the society to change. It is a top down process that starts with individual level and ends at social level (Exhibit A).

Recognizing the turbulence in the business environment that caused by Covid-19 pandemic, workers need to regard themselves as people whose value to the society and the community must be demonstrated in each successive situation they find themselves in. In the light of their contingency, individuals need to develop a mindset in changing their behavior and find an approach to their new environment and a way of managing their own life in spite of fighting the Covid-19 pandemic. Individuals must be wise to think that they are in business for themselves and that their tasks have been outsourced to them by the organization and they should act like entrepreneurs.

Organizations and government leaders will have to find creative ways to achieve much higher goals in producing products domestically rather than going outside of country to a foreign country to get products. Distribution of products should be achieved in unprecedented speed, supply chain processes should be more agile and lean, providing workers with the right operating tools and standardize business processes in era of the pandemic as they want to significantly reduce their time to market and time to volume in the form of new supply chain format.

Organizations should work in the interest of their employees and community. The wise company must work with a new way of conducting business and collaboratively with all level of society and communities to make the relation as beneficial to them as it to the individual workers as possible. But the benefits of this new work arrangement will be different from the old ones. They need to inhere in the nature of the work itself and conducting their business remotely from satellite offices and home-based.

For many IT (Information Technology) workers work in the offices should be a thing of the past. Work remotely should be adapted and they should learn how to manage their time as remote workers and act like unsupervised workers in their home-based offices. Because more and more of the organization's efforts are likely to be undertaken by on-line connectivity and remote communications, the project teams must be made up of individuals from different regions with different functional backgrounds and different countries with the capabilities of being able to switch their focus rapidly from one task to another and to work with people with very different mindsets and that does not need to be on site in person on job.

Long-term employment should be for most workers a thing of the past. The organization must recognize that they are in a difficult work environment because of a deadly virus and the impact of it. Social distancing must be enforced in order to effectively and gradually eliminate the virus both in the social events and in the workplace and in organizations. But all parties will have to make their long-term plans with the likelihood of such shifts in mind. We may overcome the

Covid-19 once the vaccine is developed, but we never can be relaxed of the next virus that could be much more deadly than the 2019.

There are 76 international companies that are in the process of developing Coronavirus vaccines. The development of Coronavirus vaccines has 11 processes that must be completed before distribution for public use.

There has been in increasing number of collaborations of the multinational pharmaceutical industry with national governments and the diversity and growing number of biotechnology companies in many countries and around the world focusing on a COVID-19 vaccine. Large pharmaceutical companies with experience in making vaccines at scale, including Johnson & Johnson, AstraZeneca, and Glaxo Smith Kline (GSK), are forming alliances with biotechnology companies, national governments and universities to accelerate progression to an effective vaccine. It is estimated that the development of the Corona vaccine should be completed by mid-year 2021. According to Novavax (September 2020) vaccines have been produced against several animal diseases caused by coronaviruses. Previous projects to develop vaccines for viruses in the family of Corona that affected humans like SARS and MERS (Middle East Respiratory Syndrome) have been tested in non-human animals. A COVID-19 vaccine is a biotechnology product intended to provide acquired immunity against coronavirus. As of September 2020, there were 321 vaccine candidates in development. However, no candidates have completed all 11 processes to develop the vaccine for Covid-19. In September, some 39 vaccine candidates were in clinical research and 33 candidates were in the 4th and 5th processes "Phase-I" and "Phase-II" trials, and 6 candidates were in 7th process "Phase-III" trials. Geopolitical issues, safety concerns for vulnerable populations and manufacturing challenges for producing billions of doses are compressing schedules to shorten the standard vaccine development timeline, in some cases combining clinical trial steps over months. A vaccine development process typically conducted sequentially over several years starting with process number 1) Identifying Antigens, 2) Produce Antigens, 3) Pre-Clinical Testing, 4) Phase-I, 5) Phase-II, 6) POC, 7) Phase-III, 8) File with FDA, 9) Registration, 10) Production; and finally 11) Distribution.

It is also important to emphasize that financial regulators should refrain from relaxing critical regulatory and supervisory safeguards during this period of the pandemic and the future deadlier viruses (Pig Flu). Weakening financial stability rules for large banking institutions would undermine the core resiliency of the financial system and increase risk to the real economy. As global financial markets become

more volatile and more economically vulnerable due to the
Covid-19 pandemic, global economy will suffer with increased
difficulties to meet financial contracts. It will be important
to act swiftly in order to avoid any disruptions in the chain of
economy growth and too much risk-averse behavior before
falling into the 2nd great depression if the actions are not taken
promptly and the financial world goes into the default. It is
important for people and organizations around the world to
always assume the worse financial and pandemic scenario like
black swan event in any events especially in the event of an
attack by a deadly virus and to plan accordingly.

The government must play a far different role in the
eliminating discrimination of any types. The government
should change the policies on public enforcement and police
brutality and injustice in addition to leading the elimination of
the Covid-19 pandemic and be ready to protect people from

any future deadly viruses. As mentioned before, governments that are less tied to the interests of the people and their health will suffer with the greater loss of lives and those countries that are more aligned with the interests of the people and social health will definitely suffer less. For example, in average 900 people have died in the United States every day since the Coronavirus has entered into the USA in 2020.

Forging a new partnership between the U.S. government and domestic organizations should be in place to first employ U.S. workers and bring down the unemployment rate in the USA. Hiring U.S. workers and replacing foreign workers especially in the IT sector should be immediate and paid attention. It is the moral responsibility of every leader in the U.S.A to hire U.S. citizen and there should not be any need for a foreign worker to be hired instead. The U.S. has enough domestic talents to take care of the IT needs replacing

3,000,000+ IT foreign workers. U.S. government should rebuild new immigration regulations and reforms INS policies in order to control the flukes of foreign workers entering to the U.S. for work.

There is more than enough talent coming from the U.S. universities to power tech companies' needs. It seems like the U.S. companies needing extraordinarily, rare and greater than doctoral scientists or engineers for their needs to fill the position. According to Insights.dice (2020) in average the U.S. companies need 10,000 new employees in different fields and it is interesting to know that the U.S. produces 1.9 million Bachelor of Art (BA) and Bachelor of Science (BS) a year, plus hundreds of thousands of Master's degree graduates plus PhDs. It seems implausible that they cannot find that number among 1.9 million graduates. It is believed that tech companies do not hefty salary to technology workers and tech companies don't dominate the category of absolute highest individual H-1B salaries overall but healthcare and medical companies tend to pay the most to foreign workers. They are more likely to source a limited number of H-1B workers, who are no doubt highly specialized in their particular subfield on medicine. Another high tech company "Microsoft" has filed for tens of thousands of H-1B visas for years before considering the U.S. workers with high education in the same field. Other high tech consulting companies like Accenture filed many H-1B visas with the salary of $96,366 a year and Capgemini pays $89,918 a year to these H-1B IT workers.

Hopefully with the current and additional executive orders from the President Trump the radical change of H-1B visas would reduce the foreign worker numbers. The H-1B visa denial rate has been increased from 6% in 2015 to 29% in 2nd quarter of 2020, that is 21% increase from 2019 and 24%

from 2018. Compare these numbers to a decade ago when the

denial rate hovered around 8%.

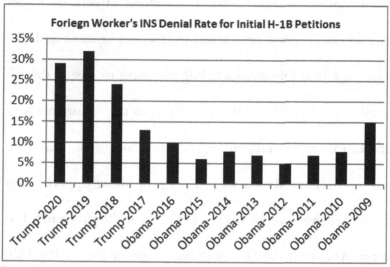

Source: Insights.dice (2020)

The president Trump has done a great job enacting

several measures to restrict the H-1B and other similar

visas climaxing with the President's recent executive order

that temporarily freezes new work visas. He may extent that

further after the election and once he runs the Whitehouse

in 2nd term. In the federal departments such as the Secretaries of Labor and Homeland Security they have taken action as appropriate and consistent with the applicable law to protect United States workers from any adverse effects on wages and working conditions caused by the employment of H-1B visa holders at job sites including measures to ensure that all employers of H-1B visa holders adhere to the requirements of the Immigration and Nationality Act. Most of the executive orders are framed as a way to open up more opportunities to unemployed workers during the Covid-19 pandemic. For most American workers wanting to get a job in the U.S. federal government and when U.S. workers are considering job specification confusion salary restraints, spares career development opportunities, inflexible education and tenure requirements, lengthy security clearance acquisition times is a tricky and rigid landscape to navigate. Federal government should not and cannot limit itself to only recruiting those with specific experience, background and certificates; instead they should draw workers from a diverse group of candidates and then offer upskilling opportunities to earn those degrees and certifications. From a practical view, recruiting talent to for the federal government can run into bureaucracy.

In April 22, 2020, President Trump issued a presidential proclamation to suspend the entry of nearly all immigrants to the United States. If the entry bans in the presidential proclamation continues, which might be for another four years if Trump is re-elected, then virtually no employment-based or family immigrants can enter America. The same goes for family of immigrants, except for the spouses and children of U.S. citizens. The proclamation action was necessary due to the high U.S. unemployment rate. Since the 1970s the U.S. has allowed thousands of foreign workers enter to the U.S. and given permanent residencies (Green Card) to 50,000 visa holders with high levels of education, age, fluency in

English, work experience, family support and demographic

considerations.

The proper public policy in response to such pandemic

with massive job loss is not protectionism, but rather assisting

individual workers to adjust to labor market changes caused

by the pandemic. Government should offer a comprehensive

array of income support through simulate programs, provide

training and retraining and eventually reemployment

services to the U.S. national workers who have lost their jobs

because of the Covid-19 pandemic. Additional assistance to

dislocated domestic workers should be available through the

Job Training Partnership Act, which is being replaced by the

Workforce Investment Act. Job search allowances should also

be provided to the U.S. workers seeking suitable employment

such as IT outside their normal commuting area.

We already have a new baseline of what's possible to do online. From working on-line to telecommute, meetings, educate, shop, medical to voting on-line and series of online games and entertainments and whole lot more. To that extent our government, institutions and social networks succeed by coming together to make the change for better collectively. As world leaders respond to the Coronavirus pandemic, they have a chance to chart a different course and make a major intervention for a healthy planet and people in it. With trillions of dollars in economic stimulus investments, they have a golden opportunity to channel significant portions of those funds to fast forward to a renewable energy economy. A transition to clean, renewable energy will seriously reduce air pollution, greenhouse gas emissions and minimize the impact of future viruses.

After every disaster something good comes out of it. It is time for a new invention and life making better stuff. Now is the time to create something real good for the current generate and our next generation as we wait for a vaccine. We should move toward with new technological innovation in the area of education on-line, eliminating on-grand classroom based teaching. Elimination of shopping centers and shopping malls and moving to cyber personalized malls. Move away from mass gathering places like churches and mosques and synagogues, worship on-line. Move away from big cities and crowed offices in downtown places and live in suburban areas where we may have a better air quality and less stress and avoiding heavy traffic. Vehicles of today will not serve tomorrow's need rather airlift vehicles and anti-gravity vehicles may do a better job of transporting. In August 28 of 2020 Japan's SkyDrive Inc. has successfully carried out a test flight of their flying car, according to the Associated Press

(AP). The flying car is drone helicopter-like propellers, while the contraption itself has no roof. We can expend that to an anti-gravity vehicle and beyond. We should move away from public bussing, underground train stations and anything that is attached to the ground, go forward toward airlift and anti-gravity vehicles for transportation. We heard a lot about anti-gravity vehicles for years but that kept secret and out of public eye for years. Forget about going back to the Moon; forget about going to Mars to build life for hand full of people. We should take care of earth problems first rather than exploring space. Get rid of discrimination and use the money and the budget that is set aside for exploring space. Use NASA budget on training masses on social order regulations and policies; reduce the hunger and poverty on earth rather than few elites moving to the orbit. It is time to look at what are actual problems on the earth not worry about the problems out in space and galaxy. Innovating solar energy in recent year is a drop in the ocean when it comes to innovating big things. Look at the innovations in Brazil and Marrakesh that are in use for years.

Brazil is the world's largest producer of ethanol fuel. Brazil government has set a policy model for all other countries to change the petrol operating vehicles to ethanol fuel. They utilized sugarcane ethanol that is the most successful alternative fuel to date. Brazil's 40-year-old ethanol fuel program is based on the most efficient agricultural technology for sugarcane cultivation in the world. All automobiles in Brazil use ethanol fuel rather than petroleum.

Morocco has launched one of the world's largest solar energy projects costing an estimated $9 billion. The aim of the project was to create 2,000 megawatts of solar generation capacity by the end of 2020. Solar power in Morocco was enabled by their government having one of the highest rates

of solar insolation in the world, about 3,600 hours per year of
sunshine generating electricity in the desert.

The U.S. has the talent and the capital to move away
from old technologies and go forward to better technological
innovations, in spite of the Covid-19 disaster. Again, according
to experts the great civilizations can only arise and merge out
of the bloody throes of societal wars.

International Business Machines, or IBM, an American
company was launched in 1911. In 1960's IBM was
dominating the IT market, Microsoft took over years later
to introduced IBM Personal Computers Operating System
(OS) for PC in 1981, Apple Corporation followed the same
and introduced the Mac in 1984. Software development for
the mainframes was done by domestic and talented American
resources, Microsoft software development took over the
personal application like word processing and other business

applications (Excel, Word). Apple initially focused on designing hardware and software for education and graphics. The software development, programming and maintenance were maintained by American workers for years till President Bill Clinton (1993-2001) took the office. The concerns over Y2K in the mid-1990s Clinton administration sets up a budget of 600,000 foreign workers to come to the U.S. from India to assist in software development for Y2K programming and fixing bugs. Ever since with the help of the Whitehouse and the support of each president thereafter, Asian-Indians have been coming to the U.S. to take over the IT industry by storm and kick out all American workers out of IT jobs. So Americans lost their jobs to Asian-Indians, Americans lost their manufacturing jobs to China and Taiwanese. Garment industry to India, Pakistan and China. What is left in the U.S. is high unemployed with Pandemic on top of it. The future of the America is not very bright the way it's going.

President Trump has fixed some of these issues by executive orders but a lot need to be done in coming years. America as a great capitalist would soon become dump ground and the backyard of other countries to dump foreign workers and pull away natural resources and steal American Intellectual Properties (IP).

According to the New York Times (2020) China steals up to $600 billion in American intellectual property (IP) every year. President Trump understands that tariffs are a powerful political tool that can and should be used to force China to pay for their crimes. Most Americans have only a fuzzy understanding of what constitutes IP. Basically, IP (Intellectual Properties) are ideas; the products of human creativity such as art, branding or inventions that can be owned and legally protected by registering copyrights, trademarks or patents. American universities are the good source of developing IP or American companies innovating new products. The American firms that initially had the blueprint and the design of those products can be out-priced and killed off the market. The IP theft costs American individuals and businesses between $225 and $600 billion annually. Most of this loss is caused by the theft of American trade secrets ($540 billion), although software piracy ($18 billion) and counterfeiting ($41 billion) are likewise significant drains. A report from the Commission on the Theft of American Intellectual Property (2017) estimated that the preponderance of this theft is committed by China and supported by Chinese government.

The U.S. Justice Department discovered a group of hackers associated with China's main intelligence service had infiltrated more than 100 companies and organizations around the world to steal intelligence, hijack their networks and extort their victims. These hacker groups, which had been predominantly targeting gaming companies, shifted to a long list of companies in the United States, Germany, Hong Kong, Japan, South Korea and Taiwan that operated in agriculture, hospitality, chemicals, manufacturing and technology whose intellectual property would assist China's official five-year plan, the nation's top-level policy blueprint. China government attempts to unlawfully advance its economy and to become the dominant global superpower through cyberattacks. According to New York Times (September 2020) the criminal computer activity and the hackers had been tracked by cyber-researchers under the group names "Advanced Persistent Threat 41", "Barium", "Winnti", "Wicked Panda" and "Panda Spider".

According to the NY Times (2020), 87% of all counterfeit goods entering America originate in either China or Hong

Kong as Chinese have done that many times in the past and is continuing to do the same at present time and at the time of reading this book. President Trump has done a very good job in this area and increased the trade tariffs for China. President Trump not only has the power to impose tariffs on China but he is morally obligated to do so. After all, the president is ultimately responsible for protecting American copyrights, trademarks, and patents both here and abroad. If tariffs help to do this, then they are justified. Both Congress and the Media misunderstood tariffs. Tariffs are not simply taxes, they are political tools. Tariffs are a means to an end that can help secure reciprocity from the U.S. trading partners and protect the U.S. IP from foreign theft.

We are entering a new age of global crisis with the Coronavirus pandemic dominating the control of the World. The road to no work for workers will collapse the fabric of global economy and disaster is within the sight. Whether that road leads to a safe haven or a terrible abyss will depend on how well civilization prepares to fight the viruses now and in the future, otherwise the end of work could spell a death sentence for civilization as we have come to know it. The end of great social economic could also signal the beginning of a great social transformation, a rebirth of the human spirit. The Coronavirus pandemic has made it clear to us that every human and planetary health is intimately interconnected.

The global pandemic has led to a significant increase in restrictions on the freedom of movement of people worldwide and worrisome reports on the misuse of emergency measures to further erode human rights and the rule of law. The prospects of a long-term global recession raise serious concerns over how these protection gaps and human rights restrictions will be addressed. Post-pandemic recovery will hopefully lead to an expansion of rights and participation of all races in public affairs so that we are more resilient to future such crises.

Lastly the Covid-19 pandemic and its social and economic impacts have created a global crisis unparalleled in the history of the world and one which requires an entire globe response to match its sheer scale and complexity. But this response, whether at the national level or international level, will be significantly weakened if it does not factor in the ways in which inequalities and injustice have made us vulnerable to the impacts of the crisis. Or, if we choose to simply repeat past policies and fail to use this moment to rebuild more equal, inclusive and resilient societies. The choice is ours to act accordingly. The future lies in our hands.

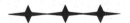

Tables and Statistics

Global Covid-19 Cases, Deaths & Recovered

Confirmed	Deaths	Recovered
36,265,982	1,057,9505	25,283,401

Source: Guardian as of October 8, 2020

Top 20 Global Covid-19 Cases, Deaths & Recovered by Country

#	Country	Confirmed	Deaths	Recovered	Death%
1	United States	7,640,553	214,985	4,958,384	3%
2	India	6,903,475	106,525	5,903,127	2%
3	Brazil	5,002,386	148,305	4,391,082	3%
4	Russia	1,260,186	22,195	1,002,207	2%
5	Peru	835,698	33,146	723,513	4%
6	Colombia	877,945	27,665	773,457	3%
7	Mexico	799,113	82,179	560,416	11%
8	South Africa	685,572	17,772	618,303	2%
9	Spain	848,040	32,695	156,376	5%
10	Argentina	601,713	12,460	448,250	2%
11	Chile	476,827	13,199	448,981	3%
12	France	428,696	31,249	90,840	7%
13	Iran	488,198	27,952	399,505	6%
14	United Kingdom	561,614	42,705	-	11%
15	Bangladesh	345,805	4,881	252,335	1%
16	Saudi Arabia	338,720	4,930	323,352	1%
17	Iraq	391,162	9,614	319,634	3%
18	Pakistan	316,386	6,508	302,683	2%
19	Turkey	330,710	8,667	290,805	2%
20	Italy	338,132	36,083	235,303	12%
	Totals	25,261,231	802,340	17,814,204	

Source: Guardian as of October 8, 2020

The USA Unemployment Rate till July 2020

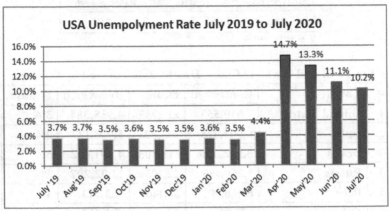

USA Unempolyment Rate July 2019 to July 2020

Source: https://www.statista.com/statistics/273909/seasonally-adjusted-monthly-unemployment-rate-in-the-us/ rate August 2020

The US unemployment rate dropped to 10.2 percent in July of 2020 from 11.1 percent in June and below market expectations of 10.5 percent, as many businesses continued to reopen and rehire employees following COVID-19 lockdowns. The number of unemployed persons fell by 1.4 million to 16.3 million. However, the jobless rate remains above the Global Financial Crisis peak of 10.0%, and more than double than February's 3.5% before the spread of the pandemic in the US. Official figures still may be far off the reality as many people are being classified as employed even though they are absent from work. (Trading Economics, 2020)

Global Unemployment Rate till March 2020

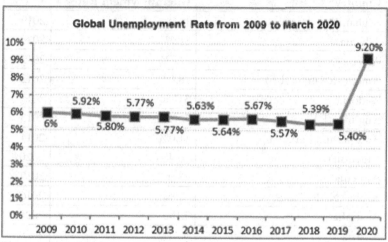

Source: www.oecd.org/economic-outlook/june-2020/

The statistic shows the global rate of unemployment from 2009 to march 2020. In the 1st quarter of 2020, the global rate of unemployment jumped to 9.2 percent.

Global Unemployment Rate by Country/Year

Country	Unemployment Rate %	Year
Afghanistan	11.1%	2019
Albania	11.9%	2020
Algeria	11.7%	2019
American Samoa (US)	18.0%	2012
Andorra	3.7%	2017
Anguilla (UK)	7.8%	2013
Antigua and Barbuda	11.0%	2014
Argentina	10.4%	2020
Armenia	18.9%	2019
Aruba (Netherlands)	7.7%	2016
Australia	7.1%	2020
Austria	5.4%	2020
Azerbaijan	5.5%	2019
Bahrain	0.7%	2019
Bangladesh	4.2%	2019
Barbados	10.3%	2019
Belarus	4.6%	2019
Belgium	5.4%	2020
Belize	6.4%	2019
Bermuda	7.0%	2017
Bhutan	2.3%	2019
Bolivia	3.5%	2019
Bosnia and Herzegovina	18.4%	2019
Botswana	18.2%	2019
Brazil	12.2%	2020
British Virgin Islands (UK)	2.9%	2019

Global Unemployment Rate by Country/Year

Country	Unemployment Rate %	Year
Brunei	9.1%	2019
Bulgaria	9.0%	2020
Burma	1.6%	2019
Cambodia	0.7%	2019
Cameroon	3.4%	2019
Canada	12.3%	2019
Cape Verde	12.2%	2019
Cayman Islands (UK)	3.5%	2019
Central African Republic	3.7%	2019
Chad	1.9%	2019
Chile	11.2%	2020
China	5.9%	2020
Cocos Islands (Australia)	6.7%	2011
Colombia	19.8%	2020
Comoros	4.3%	2019
Cook Islands	13.1%	2005
Costa Rica	12.4%	2020
Croatia	9.5%	2020
Cuba	1.6%	2019
Cyprus	8.9%	2020
Czech Republic	3.4%	2020
Denmark	5.0%	2020
Djibouti	10.3%	2019
Dominica	23.0%	2016
Dominican Republic	5.8%	2019
East Timor	4.5%	2019

Global Unemployment Rate by Country/Year

Country	Unemployment Rate %	Year
Ecuador	4.9%	2019
Egypt	7.7%	2020
El Salvador	4.1%	2019
Equatorial Guinea	4.1%	2019
Estonia	6.0%	2020
Eswatini	22.1%	2019
European Union	6.7%	2020
Faroe Islands (Denmark)	0.9%	2019
Fiji	4.1%	2019
Finland	10.6%	2020
France	8.1%	2019
French Polynesia (France)	12.1%	2019
Gabon	20.0%	2019
Georgia	12.8%	2019
Germany	3.9%	2020
Ghana	4.3%	2019
Gibraltar (UK)	1.0%	2016
Greece	14.4%	2020
Greenland (Denmark)	6.8%	2017
Grenada	24%	2017
Guam (US)	4.5%	2017
Guatemala	2.5%	2019
Guernsey (UK)	1.0%	2018
Guyana	4.3%	2019
Honduras	5.4%	2019
Hong Kong	5.9%	2020

Global Unemployment Rate by Country/Year

Country	Unemployment Rate %	Year
Hungary	4.1%	2020
Iceland	4.5%	2020
India	8.5%	2020
Indonesia	5.0%	2020
Iran	11.4%	2019
Iraq	12.8%	2019
Ireland	5.3%	2020
Isle of Man	3.0%	2020
Israel	4.2%	2020
Italy	7.8%	2020
Jamaica	8.0%	2019
Japan	2.6%	2020
Jersey (UK)	1.6%	2020
Jordan	14.7%	2019
Kazakhstan	4.8%	2020
Kenya	2.6%	2019
Kiribati	30.6%	2010
Kosovo	25.9%	2019
Kuwait	2.2%	2019
Kyrgyzstan	6.3%	2019
Laos	0.6%	2019
Latvia	9.8%	2020
Lebanon	6.2%	2019
Lesotho	23.4%	2019
Libya	18.6%	2019
Liechtenstein	1.5%	2019

Global Unemployment Rate by Country/Year

Country	Unemployment Rate %	Year
Lithuania	9.3%	2020
Luxembourg	7.7%	2020
Macau (China)	2.2%	2019
Malaysia	5.0%	2020
Mali	6.1%	2019
Malta	4.0%	2020
Marshall Islands	36.0%	2006
Mauritania	9.5%	2019
Mauritius	6.7%	2019
Mayotte (France)	30.0%	2019
Mexico	3.3%	2019
Federated States of Micronesia	16.2%	2019
Moldova	4.1%	2019
Monaco	2.0%	2019
Mongolia	6.0%	2019
Montenegro	18.2%	2019
Montserrat(UK)	5.6%	2017
Morocco	10.5%	2020
Mozambique	3.2%	2019
Namibia	20.3%	2019
Nauru	23.0%	2011
Nepal	11.4%	2019
Netherlands	3.6%	2020
Netherlands Antilles (Netherlands)	21.2%	2019
New Caledonia (France)	12.8%	2019
New Zealand	4.2%	2020

Global Unemployment Rate by Country/Year

Country	Unemployment Rate %	Year
Nicaragua	6.5%	2019
Nigeria	23.1%	2018
North Korea	2.7%	2019
North Macedonia	17.8%	2019
Northern Mariana Islands (US)	11.2%	2010
Norway	8.8%	2020
Oman	2.7%	2019
Pakistan	4.5%	2019
Palau	1.7%	2015
Palestine	25.3%	2019
Panama	3.9%	2019
Papua New Guinea	2.5%	2019
Paraguay	5.7%	2019
Peru	13.1%	2020
Philippines	17.7%	2019
Poland	3.0%	2019
Portugal	5.5%	2019
Puerto Rico (US)	8.8%	2020
Qatar	0.1%	2019
Romania	5.2%	2020
Russia	6.1%	2020
Rwanda	13.1%	2020
Saint Helena (UK)	14%	1998
Saint Kitts and Nevis	5.1%	2006
Saint Lucia	15.7%	2006
Saint Pierre and Miquelon (France)	8.7%	2015

Global Unemployment Rate by Country/Year

Country	Unemployment Rate %	Year
Saint Vincent and the Grenadines	18.8%	2008
San Marino	8.0%	2017
Saudi Arabia	5.7%	2019
Senegal	6.6%	2019
Serbia	9.5%	2019
Sierra Leone	4.4%	2019
Singapore	2.4%	2020
Slovakia	6.5%	2020
Slovenia	4.8%	2020
Somalia	11.4%	2019
South Africa	30.1%	2020
South Korea	4.5%	2020
Spain	14.5%	2020
Sri Lanka	4.5%	2019
Sudan	16.5%	2019
Suriname	7.3%	2019
Sweden	8.5%	2020
Switzerland	4.4%	2020
Syria	8.4%	2019
Taiwan	4.1%	2020
Tajikistan	11.0%	2019
Thailand	1.0%	2020
Tanzania	2.0%	2019
Tonga	2.0%	2019
Trinidad and Tobago	2.7%	2019
Tunisia	15.1%	2019

Global Unemployment Rate by Country/Year

Country	Unemployment Rate %	Year
Turkey	13.2%	2020
Turkmenistan	3.9%	2019
Ukraine	8.6%	2020
United Arab Emirates	2.3%	2019
United Kingdom	3.8%	2020
United States	11.1%	2020
Uruguay	9.7%	2020
Uzbekistan	8.9%	2019
Vanuatu	4.4%	2019
Venezuela	8.8%	2019
Vietnam	2.2%	2019
U.S. Virgin Islands (US)	8.7%	2019
Wallis and Futuna (France)	8.8%	2019
Yemen	12.9%	2019
Zambia	11.4%	2019
Zimbabwe	5.0%	2019

Source: https://en.wikipedia.org/w/index.php?title=List_of_countries_by_unemployment
_rate&action=edit&section=1 (2020)

Charts and Graphics

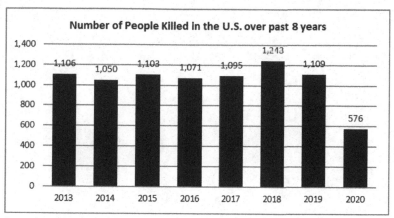

Source: mappingpoliceviolence.org (March, 2020)

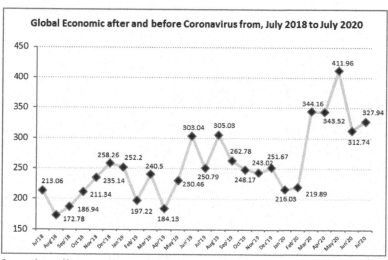

Source: https://www.statista.com/statistics....... (Aug, 2020)

Exhibit A

Top-Down Change Process

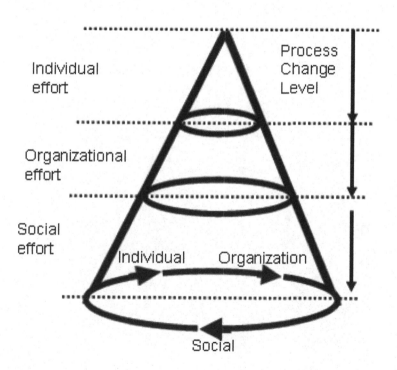

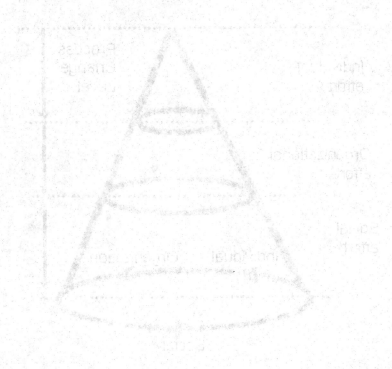

References

ABC News (2020). "Some leaders use pandemic to sharpen tools against critics".

Adolf Hitler, Mein Kampf (English Translation, Boston 1971) p. 55.

Adolf Hitler, Mein Kampf, p. 204.

Aislelabs (2020). "How Retailers Globally are Responding to Coronavirus by Aislelabs".

Aislelabs (2020). "How Shopping Centres Globally are Responding to Coronavirus by Aislelabs".

Al Jazeera (2020). "Global hunger could double due to coronavirus pandemic: UN".

Al Jazeera (2020). "Half the world's workers face losing their jobs, says ILO".

Al Jazeera (2020). "Trump, aides flirt with China lab coronavirus conspiracy theory".

Al Omran A & Kerr S (2020). "Saudi Arabia bans Mecca pilgrimages over coronavirus fears". Financial Times.

Antisemitismus der Vernunft. In: Adolf Hitler, Gutachten über den Antisemitismus (1919) erstellt im Auftrag seiner militärischen Vorgesetzten'. Included in: Maser, Werner, Hitlers Briefe und Notizen (Düsseldorf 1973).

Aron, R. (1968). <u>Main currents in sociological thought</u>. New York: Dover, 36.

Associated Press (2020). "Coronavirus brings entertainment world to a standstill".

Associated Press (2020). "Countries Evaluate Evacuation of Citizens Amid Wuhan Coronavirus Panic".

Australian Government (2020). "Coronavirus (COVID-19) information for Australian travellers".

Bangkok Post, (2020). Online News

BBC News (2020). "China McDonald's apologizes for Guangzhou ban on black people".

BBC News (2020). "Collapsed Flybe: 'Do not travel to the airport'".

BBC News (2020). "Coronavirus: Anti-Lockdown Protests Grow Across US".

BBC News (2020). "Coronavirus: Could African countries cope with an outbreak?".

BBC News (2020). "Coronavirus: US workers seeking jobless aid near 40 million".

BBC News (2020). "Coronavirus: World risks 'biblical' famines due to pandemic—UN".

BBC News (2020). "US oil prices turn negative as demand dries up".

BBC News (2020), "Mystery pneumonia virus probed in China". 3 January 2020.

Beinart, Peter (2012). "The Crisis of Zionism"

Brigitte Hamann, Hitler's Vienna: A Portrait of the Tyrant as a Young Man (New York, NY and Oxford: Oxford University Press, 1999), p. 356-359.

Blanchflower, Danny (2004). "Well-being over time in Britain and the USA DG Journal of public economics". 88 (7-8). 1359-1386, 2004

Burke, D (2020). "What churches, mosques and temples are doing to fight the spread of coronavirus". CNN.

CDC (Centers for Disease Control and Prevention), (2020)

Chan JF, Yuan S, Kok KH, To KK, Chu H, Yang J, et al. (2020). "A familial cluster of pneumonia associated with the 2019 novel coronavirus indicating person-to-person transmission: a study of a family cluster". Lancet. 395 (10223): 514–523.

Cherney, Mike ; **Craymer**, Lucy (2020). "You've Got Mail ... Finally: The Pandemic Is Jamming Up the World's Post".

China News, (2020). Online News

Clamp, R (5 March 2020). "Coronavirus and the Black Death: spread of misinformation and xenophobia shows we haven't learned from our past".

Clamp, (2020)

CMGPPI (2017). "Community Mitigation Guidelines to Prevent Pandemic Influenza—United States, 2017".

CNBC, (2020). Online News

CNBC, Scipioni, Jade (18 March 2020). "Why there will soon be tons of toilet paper and what food may be scarce, according to supply chain experts".

CNN (2020). "Hungarian parliament votes to let Viktor Orban rule by decree in wake of coronavirus pandemic".

CNN News (2020). "Broadway theaters to suspend all performances because of coronavirus".

CNN Politics (2020). Online News

Comte, A. (1858). The positive philosophy, trans. Harriet Martineau. New York: Calvin Blanchard, 25-26.

Comte, A. (1974). Considerations on the spiritual power. In Ronald Fletcher (ed.).

Connecticut Mirror, (2020)

Courtney, Joe. the Congressman of Connecticut (2020)

Debate.org, (2020). Online News

Deutsche Bank, (2020)

Die "Judenzählung" von 1916. Deutsches Historisches Museum, Berlin. https://www.dhm.de/lemo/kapitel/ erster-weltkrieg/innenpolitik/judenzaehlung-1916. html [13 November 2018].

Drucker, P. (1999). "Self-Assessment Tool"

EU CDPC, (2020)

Fariza, I (2020). "La pandemia amenaza con dejar entre 14 y 22 millones de personas más en pobreza extrema en Latinoamérica". EL PAÍS (in Spanish).

Federal Reserve Administration (2020)

Federation for American Immigration Reform, (2020)

Fox News (2020). "Netherlands becomes latest country to reject China-made coronavirus test kits, gear".

France 24 (2020). "Covid-19 in Madagascar: The president's controversial 'miracle cure'".

France 24 (2020). "Iran's Khamenei refuses US help to fight coronavirus, citing conspiracy theory".

France 24 (2020). "Violence flares in tense Paris suburbs as heavy-handed lockdown stirs 'explosive cocktail'".

Gambrell, J. (2020). "Iran news agencies report Friday prayers canceled in Tehran". The Washington Post & Associated Press.

Gambrell, J. (2020). "Shiite Hardliners in Iran Storm 2 Shrines That Were Closed to Stop Coronavirus Spread". Time & Associated Press.

Garcia S, Albaghdadi MS, Meraj PM, Schmidt C, Garberich R, **Jaffer** FA, et al. (2020). "Reduction in ST-Segment Elevation Cardiac Catheterization Laboratory Activations in the United States during COVID-19 Pandemic". Journal of the ACC.

Gardner, M. J. (1995). Worker displacement: a decade of change. Monthly Labor Review.

Ghaffary, S. & **Heilweil,** R. (2020). "How tech companies are scrambling to deal with coronavirus hoaxes". Vox.

Gisanddata.maps.arcgis.com (2020). "Operations Dashboard for ArcGIS".

Global Times (2020). "Chinese medical supplies' 'quality concerns' overblown".

Haberman, M. **Martin** J (2020). "Trump's Re-election Chances Suddenly Look Shakier". The New York Times.

Hadden, J. (2020). "Over 20,000 people have signed a petition to cancel SXSW over coronavirus worries". Business Insider.

Herman, Edward (1999). "After the Cataclysm"

Hipple, S. (1997). Worker displacement in an expanding economy. Monthly Labor Review.

Hipple, S. (1999). Ongoing labor market strength reduces worker displacement. Monthly Labor Review.

INS (2020). Online News

Kang, D (2020). "The shunned: People from virus-hit city tracked, quarantined".

Kennedy, Merrit (2020). "WHO Declares Coronavirus Outbreak A Global Health Emergency". NPR.

Kubler-Ross, E. (1969). <u>On death and dying.</u> New York: Collier Books, 41-43, 64-98, 342-343.

Kubler-Ross, E. (1983). <u>On Children and death</u>. New York: MacMillan Publishing Company, 61.

Kuo, L, **Davidson** H (29 March 2020). "'They see my blue eyes then jump back'—China sees a new wave of xenophobia". The Guardian.

LA Times, (2020). Online News

Letters in Applied Microbiology, (2020)

Lewin, K. (1935). <u>A dynamic theory of personality.</u> New York: McGraw-Hill Book Company, 80-83.

Luna, F (2020). "DOH sets aside inaccurate donated test kits, assures public only quality tests are used". PhilStar Global.

McFarling, (2020)

Migrant Rights (2020). "The COVID-19 crisis is fueling more racist discourse towards migrant workers in the Gulf".

MSN News, (2020). www.msn.com

National Review (2020). "Will Iran's Regime Survive Coronavirus?".

New York Post, (2020). Online News

News.cgtn.com/news, (2020). Online News

Novel Coronavirus Pneumonia Emergency Response Epidemiology Team (February 2020). "[The epidemiological characteristics of an outbreak of 2019 novel coronavirus diseases (COVID-19) in China]". Zhonghua Liu Xing Bing Xue Za Zhi Zhonghua Liuxingbingxue Zazhi (in Chinese). 41 (2): 145–151.

NPIs, (2020). Online News

Nsikan, Akpan (2020). "Coronavirus spikes outside China show travel bans aren't working". National Geographic.

OSHA (Occupational Safety and Health Administration), (2020)

Oswald, Andrew (1994). "Unhappiness and Unemployment". The Economic Journal 104 (424). 648-659

Pascoe, (2009). Online News

Patriot Journal, (2020). Online News

Reed, S (2020). "OPEC Scrambles to React to Falling Oil Demand From China". The New York Times.

Report, (2020). Online News

Republican House of Senate, (2020)

Reuters (2020). "Coronavirus scare: Complete list of airlines suspending flights". India Today.

Reuters (2020). "Brazil suffers record coronavirus deaths, Trump mulls travel ban".

Reuters (2020). "Trump: Asian-Americans not responsible for virus, need protection".

Reuters (2020). "U.S. sanctions 'severely hamper' Iran coronavirus fight, Rouhani says".

Rifkin, J. (1995). The end of work: technology, jobs and your future. New York: Putnam Book. Pp.7, 11,101, 118,292-293.

Sanal, Basin (2020). "Turkey ranks third worldwide in supplying medical aid".

Saul, **Loeb**/AFP, (2020)

South China Morning Post (SCMP), (2020). Online News

Spencer, H. (1851). Social statics. London: Chapman, 19-23.

Spencer, H. (1874). The study of sociology. New York: D. Appleton & Company, 401- 404.

Spencer, H. (1955). The principles of psychology, 2nd edn, 2 vols. London: Longmans, 500-502.

Spencer, H. (1969). Principles of sociology. London: MacMillan, 29.

Spencer, H. (1988). Evolutionary theory. American Journal of Sociology 93, 154.

Spencer, Herbert (1874). "The Study of Sociology". NY: D. Appleton & Company. P. 401

Stuff Company (2020). "Air New Zealand flight with kiwi evacuees departs Wuhan".

Taleb, Nassim Nicholas (2004). nvestopedia; https://www. investopedia.com/terms/b/blackswan.asp

Tavernise S, Oppel Jr RA (23 March 2020). "Spit On, Yelled At, Attacked: Chinese-Americans Fear for Their Safety". The New York Times.

Tempo News, (2020) Brazilian Online News

The Balance, (2020). Online News

The Brussels Times (2020). "Coronavirus: Flanders gets 100,000 unusable masks".

The Guardian (2020). "Authoritarian leaders may use Covid-19 crisis to tighten their grip".

The Guardian (2020). "Spain calls for action from Europe as daily death toll rises again".

The New York Times (2020), "A List of What's Been Canceled Because of the Coronavirus".

The New York Times (2020). "Coronavirus Travel Restrictions, Across the Globe".

The New York Times (2020). "For Autocrats, and Others, Coronavirus Is a Chance to Grab Even More Power".

The New York Times (2020). "God Will Protect Us".

The Straits Times (2020). "Asia cracks down on coronavirus 'fake news'".

The Times News (2020). "Coronavirus Forces Families to Make Painful Childcare Decisions".

The Wall Street Journal (2020). "Italians Are Being Treated as a Risk Abroad Over Coronavirus".

The Wall Street Journal (2020). "Not Enough Doctors in Daegu: As Virus Cases Rise, South Korea's Response Is criticized".

Top10.com, (2020). Online News

Torero, Maximo (2020). "How to Stop a Looming Food Crisis". Foreign Policy.

Toynbee, A. (1957). <u>Study of history</u>. New York: Oxford University, 283.

Toynbee, A. (1961). <u>Reconsiderations</u>. New York: Oxford University Press, 198.

U.S. Bureau of Labor Statistics (2020).

U.S. Census Bureau, (2020)

U.S. Centers for Disease Control and Prevention (CDC) (2020). "Coronavirus Disease 2019 (COVID-19)".

U.S. Centers for Disease Control and Prevention (CDC) (2020). "COVID-19 Information for Travel".

U.S. Centers for Disease Control and Prevention (CDC) (2020). "Prevention & Treatment".

U.S. Equal Employment Opportunity Commission (EEOC), (2020)

UNESCO (2020), "COVID-19 Educational Disruption and Response".

UNESCO (2020). "Adverse consequences of school closures".

UNESCO (2020). "Distance learning solutions".

USA Today, (2020).

Views of CGTN, (2020). Online News

Webster's New World Dictionary of America (1988). New York: Simon & Schuster, 889.

White House, (2020). Online News

WHO (2019), "Statement on the second meeting of the International Health Regulations (2005) Emergency Committee regarding the outbreak of novel coronavirus (2019-nCoV)".

WHO (2020). "Advice for public".

WHO (2020). "Coronavirus disease (COVID-19) advice for the public: Myth busters".

WHO (2020). "Novel Coronavirus". World Health Organization (WHO).

WHO, (2020). "WHO Director-General's remarks at the media briefing on 2019-nCoV on 11 February 2020".

WHO Report (2020). "Novel Coronavirus(2019-nCoV): Situation Report-10" (PDF). World Health Organization.

Wikipedia (2020). "Racial Discrimination".

World Health Organization (2020). "WHO Director-General's opening remarks at the media briefing on COVID-19 – 11 March 2020".

World-o-Meter, (2020). Online News

Xiao, B (2020). "'No-one in the family knows what to do': Over 100 Australian children trapped in Wuhan coronavirus area". ABC News.

Xie, H (2020). "Xi stresses winning people's war against novel coronavirus". Xinhua News Agency. Xi Jinping, general secretary of the Communist Party of China Central Committee.

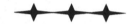

Acronym

ANTIFA – Anti-Fascist Political Activist

ARA - Anti-Racist Action

CDC – Center of Disease Control and Prevention

COBOL - Common Business-Oriented Language

DoL – Department of Labor

Covid-19 - **Co**rona **V**irus **D**isease of the year 2019)

FDA – Food & Drug Administration

GDP – Gross Domestic Product

GFC - Global Financial Crisis

H-1B Visas – particular type of visa that is used in the United States as a visa to allow foreign citizens to temporarily work in the United States

H-2B visas - permits employers to temporarily hire nonimmigrants to perform nonagricultural labor or services in the United States.

INS – Immigration and Naturalization Service

IRS - Internal Revenue Service

IT – Information Technology

L1 Visas – Non Immigrant Visa valid for a relatively short amount of time, from three months (Iran) to five years (India, Japan, Germany), based on a reciprocity schedule

NATO - North Atlantic Treaty Organization

NASA - National Aeronautics and Space Administration

OPEC - Organization of the Petroleum Exporting Countries

OS – Operating System

OSHA - Occupational Safety and Health Administration

PHEIC - Public Health Emergency of International Concern

PPE – Personal Protective Equipment

SARS - Severe Acute Respiratory Syndrome

TVA - Tennessee Valley Authority

R&D – Research and Development

UN - United Nation

UNECLA - United Nations Economic Commission for Latin America)

USA – United States of America

USCIS – U.S. Citizenship and Immigration Services

Y2K – Year 2000

WHO - World Health Organization

Wi-Fi – Wireless Fidelity

WTI - West Texas Intermediate

WW2 – World War 2

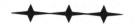

Printed in the United States
By Bookmasters